A BEGINNER'S GUIDE TO SUSTAINABLE PLANT-BASED WEIGHT-LOSS

A DIET SOLUTION FOR WOMEN TO LOSE WEIGHT, KEEP IT OFF, AND IMPROVE HEALTH

SHANE CORBITT

CONTENTS

Just For You

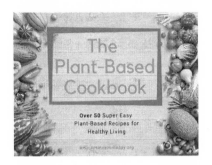

A Free Gift to My Readers
Over 50 Plant-Based Recipes. Download and Start Eating
Healthy Today!

www.createyourhappy.org/cookbook

INTRODUCTION

 "Dieting is the only game where you win when you lose"

— KARL LAGERFELD

You cannot talk about nutrition and drop the phrase "plant-based" in this twenty-first-century era. Plant-based diets are increasingly becoming trendy, to say the least. This is because this type of diet comes with remarkable success in addressing weight-gain issues and improving the overall health of individuals. It is also a more efficient option when it comes to sustaining the environment. For this reason and more, many people all over the world are turning to plant-based diets.

Why Plant-Based Diets?

There are many reasons why plant-based diets have gained so much ground in the past years. One of such reasons is an increased awareness of the health benefits of adopting plant-based diets. Greens are known for improving cardiovascular and brain health. Promoting weight loss also reduces the risk of other diseases such as heart disease and diabetes. A plant-based diet also enhances the functionality of your digestive system. You can save yourself from the hustle of having to constantly deal with issues such as constipation, overeating, and compromised absorption. Nutritionally, a diet that excludes plants is incomplete. Plants host an abundance of nutrients that you might be unable to find in meats and other animal-based foods.

Moreover, plants don't contain most of the nutrients that negatively affect your health. You cannot find saturated fatty acids in plants, for example. This means that going plant-based increases the chances of being healthier overall.

Some prefer diets that are plant-based for ethical reasons. The main idea is to avoid consuming meats and dairy products with the notion that doing this is more moral. Therefore, the ethical reasons for adopting diets hinged on plants are based on "animal empathy." Animal-based diets may involve testing products using animals, which is less likely to happen with plant-based foods. Even if plants are also processed, animals' pain before having the meat on your plate could cause concern. Interestingly, it has been reported that people whose orientation toward plant-based foods is due to ethical concerns have a higher probability of being loyal to the diet for longer (Scott-Thomas, 2015).

Plant-Based Diets and Celebrities

Many celebrities have turned to meatless food as the central part of their diet. This is how popular this type of diet has become. Let's briefly look at some of such celebrities:

- **Venus Williams:** Venus Williams is a famous tennis

player. Initially, she adopted the vegan diet for health reasons. Venus was diagnosed with Sjögren's syndrome, which is an autoimmune disease. This condition compromises the production of moisture in glands like tear and saliva-producing glands. This is what Venus had to say to the *Health*, "Once I started, I fell in love with the concept of fueling your body in the best way possible. Not only does it help me on the court, but I feel like I'm doing the right thing for me" (Vogel, 2021).

- **Zac Efron:** Zac Efron is a prominent actor who started his vegan journey in 2018. From Zac's experience with the plant-based diet, he emphasizes that the diet has been excellent for his exercises and everyday routines. While talking to *Teen Vogue*, Zac said, "I've been experimenting with eating purely vegan. That's completely changed the way that my body works, and the way that I metabolize food, the way it turns into energy, the way that I sleep" (Nast, 2018).

- **Ariana Grande:** Ariana Grande is a pop star who is an "animal fanatic." Her love for animals forms the foundation for why she swears by the complete vegan diet—There is no option B for her when it comes to diet. According to Ariana, a whole food diet can increase your lifespan, in addition to making you a happier person overall. During her interview with the *Daily Mirror*, Ariana said, "It is tricky dining out, but I just stick to what I know—veggies, fruit, and salad, then when I get home, I'll have something else" (Gilmour, 2018).

- **Beyonce and Jay Z:** Beyonce's love with the plant-based diet began as an "experiment." Together with her husband Jay Z, Beyonce took up a 22-day challenge of eating a completely meatless diet. Having loved the results of their 'challenge,' Beyonce went on to publicly announce her newly-adopted diet on Instagram. The singer wrote, "44 days until Coachella!! Vegan Time!! Click the link in my bio to join me!" (Vogel, 2021).

- **Liam Hemsworth:** Liam Hemsworth's story reflects the power of association in developing certain habits like eating patterns and food preferences. His friends went vegan first, and that was enough motivation to get the Australian actor started with this type of diet.

Get the Best out of Plant-Based Diets

You might have tried various other diets recommended for you by friends, colleagues, family, or the internet, all to no avail. This situation is not unique to you alone; I also had my own share of the experience. There are so many diets out there that are linked to having cosmetic properties, aiding weight loss, being energizing, and improving general health. After trying them, I realized that the benefits associated with the diets were only theoretical. All this happened before I started the plant-based diet. With a meatless diet, you will never go wrong in terms of health, nutrition, self-esteem, and higher energy levels.

Weight loss can be a significant cause for concern, especially to women. This is because it affects your shape and health, thereby ultimately fueling low self-confidence. Unfortunately, with the increased variety and availability of food out there, it is difficult to make the right choices with regard to what you should consume. This is the primary cue for weight gain. If you have tried other diets before, you might have noticed that most of them are challenging to stick to, which is the reason why you would quit before getting your desired body shape.

Did some of the diets that you've tried seem to work during the first few days or weeks as you dropped some pounds? You then wondered why you suddenly started gaining weight again? This is a very common scenario with many diets that come and go. Usually, it is because diets are too complicated to keep up with on a long-term basis. Such diets are often referred to as fad diets, and I call them "come and go" diets. The plant-based diet that is presented in this book cannot be compared with these fad diets. It is here to stay because you can quickly adapt and sustain it for a lifetime without making your body feel deprived.

Most diets out there are designed in a way that makes it difficult for your body to get used to them. Most of them are strict on a few foods, which make them monotonous and boring. Contrastingly, the plant-based diet is laced with variety, so it is relatively easier to stick to. Therefore, if you have been looking for a sustainable diet that can address your weight concerns for a lifetime, you have just reached your final stop — plant-based diet it is!

This book will enlighten you on the important things that you need to know concerning the plant-based diet. It will explain the role of the plant-based diet in aiding weight loss and other health benefits. Quite often, the best way to do a thing is by avoiding specific actions or behaviors. This is why this book will focus on the dos associated with food consumption and look at the don'ts. To help you add some variety and fun to your plant-based diet, this book will also provide you with tips for making your lifetime eating experience the best that it can be. Not only that, this book is furnished with recipes for all meals and for snacking. Therefore, with this book in your hands, you have a complete package and guide that will trigger and maintain the endless passion for plant-based foods.

Meet the Author

Shane Corbitt is an expert in nutrition and weight loss. Shane is passionate and enthusiastic about sharing his knowledge of the proper strategies that aid weight loss. Having been studying plant-based nutrition and how it contributes to appropriate weight loss for years, Shane is in an excellent position to provide readers with authentic information about plant-based diet interventions for weight loss. He desires to provide others with practical and applicable information that will see them achieve their desired weight goals.

Apart from his academic knowledge, Shane experienced what it's like to try many diets without getting the desired results — the pain, frustration, hopelessness, and boredom, you name it. This is part of what motivated Shane to develop a plant-based diet plan that has proven very successful for women of a wide range of ages. He's worked tirelessly to collect suitable recipes and information for women to reach their weight goals. In summary, Shane is authoring this "long-awaited" book because he believes in the power of plant-based diets and how important it is to find the proper diet that works.

THE ESSENCE OF PLANT-BASED DIETS

A plant-based diet is described as the emphasized consumption of plant-centered products. It is also referred to as sustainable eating because it is concerned about healthy and environmentally friendly food. This diet focuses on fresh and whole plant-based ingredients while minimizing the consumption of refined food. Legumes, whole grains, nuts, seeds, fruits, herbs, spices, and vegetables are some examples of plant-based ingredients. A plant-based diet limits or eliminates your intake of all products of animal origin, including fish, cheese, eggs, and milk. This chapter will enlighten you on foundational aspects surrounding plant-based diets. To begin with, the next section will explore the reasons why a plant-based diet is appealing.

Why Choose a Plant-Based Diet?

People have various reasons, motives, and goals why they opt for plant-based diets. These reasons range from personal beliefs to those of group affiliations. Here are some of the considerations that trigger people into following diets that are based on plants:

- **Weight-loss goals:** A plant-based diet is an attractive option to most people who want to lose weight.

- **Medicinal purposes:** The diet is also popular for its incredible medicinal properties that help your body fight and prevent diseases.

- **Upholding animal rights:** Some people make this decision for animal welfare because they believe that all animals have the right to life and freedom rather than their consumption is an infringement of such privilege.

- **Religious doctrines:** Members of Islam, Buddhism, and Jainism strongly believe that abstaining from meat shows kindness, mercy, and respect to animals. Christianity and Judaism are inspired by Bible scriptures that emphasize the types of food that they should eat. Hinduism accepts the diet as a spiritual practice toward the "sacred cow." In ancient India, the survival of farmers was dependent on cow products. They used cow milk, curd, and ghee as food, while dung and urine were used as fertilizers to cultivate crops. Hence, the cow was their symbol of prosperity and life.

- **Allergies from animal products:** Some people suffer from alpha-gal syndrome because they are highly allergic to red meat and animal products, while others are lactose intolerant.

- **Differences in taste preferences:** Some people simply don't enjoy animal-based products. Their taste buds fancy a plant-based diet.

- **Environmental considerations:** Animal agriculture has been attributed to a number of adverse environmental impacts. These include greenhouse gas emissions, and large amounts of water and land used when rearing livestock. This gives people an urge to convert to a sustainable plant-based diet.

- **Proving the sustenance point:** Other people want to prove a point that humans don't have to rely on animal products for survival because you can certainly obtain all essential nutrients from a plant-based diet.

The "Must-Know" Facts About Plant-Based Diets

There have been spotlight debates on the protein content of plant-based diets, considering that there is restricted meat intake. Plant-based diet practitioners also highlighted that their diet is cheaper than meat products, which are usually more expensive to purchase. Some participants in the debate also stressed that plant-based diets are insufficient in providing other adequate essential nutrients such as vitamin B12, which are required by the human body. In this section, we will delve deeper into the facts around these debates.

Absolutely No Meat!

Depending on personal preferences, a plant-based diet abstains from meat intake and any animal-centered products at different levels. It's either total exclusion, or occasional inclusion of animal-based food is involved. Therefore, there are different categories of a plant-based diet, as highlighted below.

A Vegetarian Diet

Vegetarians focus their meals on plant-based ingredients, but they also include dairy products, eggs, and seafood. They exclude all poultry and meat. There are different categories of vegetarian diets based on the animal ingredients that they eat. These are:

- **A Lacto-vegetarian diet:** This diet includes honey and dairy products to their diet while excluding meat and eggs.

- **An Ovo-vegetarian diet** includes eggs and honey to their plant-based diet but excludes seafood, fish, and meat.

- **A Lacto-ovo-vegetarian diet:** This diet includes eggs, honey, and dairy products to their diet but with no meat.

- **A Pescatarian diet:** This diet includes seafood, fish, honey, eggs, and dairy products to their diet. However, they exclude poultry and beef from their meals.

A Vegan Diet

Vegans abstain from eating any animal by-products like eggs, dairy, honey, and absolutely no meat. The diet allows the consumption of processed or refined plant-based food in addition to whole food.

A Whole Food Plant-Based Diet

Plant-based foods are eaten in their whole form while restricting any oils, processed, or refined food consumption. This is flexible on meat restrictions compared to the other types because some might occasionally add meat to their meals. However, it still limits the intake of animal by-products as the general idea of a plant-based diet.

The Mediterranean Diet

The diet is high in plant-based food. It includes consuming moderate amounts of meat, seafood, fish, eggs, poultry, and dairy products.

Plant-Based Diets Help You Save Money

Converting from meat-based meals to a plant-based diet significantly cuts your grocery budget. Sous Vide Guy revealed that people who eat meat-based meals spent approximately $23 more than vegetarians or vegans (Exploring Opinions on Plant-Based Eating, n.d.). This is because animal by-products are expensive and cost at least $3 more than plant food of the same quantity.

Animal-based foods are also expensive to produce, considering the money needed to rear livestock and process and deliver meat, eggs, and dairy products. As a result, meat is deemed luxurious, especially by low-income households, while a plant-based diet is pocket-friendly. Thus, choosing to munch on plant-based protein food is an excellent strategy for enriching your body with nutrients on a cheap budget.

A Variety of Food Options

Transitioning to a plant-based diet provides you with an array of tasty and nourishing food options. It doesn't limit your nutritional requirements simply because they are meatless. Food options in a plant-oriented diet come in six groups, nourishing and satisfying your dietary needs at all levels. These are:

- **Fruits:** Fruits are nutritious and packed with vitamin C and A, fiber, potassium, folate, and magnesium. They are also filled with plant-protective chemicals such as polyphenols. These chemicals, also called phytochemicals because they come from plants, have antioxidant and anti-inflammatory properties that your body utilizes to combat diseases. Apples, bananas, blueberries, avocados, and citrus fruits are some examples of good fruits.

- **Vegetables** generally supply calcium, magnesium, zinc, and vitamins A, B, C, and K. They also possess flavonoids, which are a type of phytochemical. Flavonoids in celery help the body fight inflammation and the damage of cells caused by oxidation.

- **Whole grains** consist of staple foods that provide plant-based protein, zinc, fiber, iron, magnesium, vitamins B and E. They also contain phytochemicals that boost your immune system. Whole grains include amaranth, wild rice, oats, quinoa, and buckwheat.

- **Legumes** are inexpensive and jammed with nutrients, such as protein, zinc, fiber, iron, magnesium, phosphorus, selenium, and folate. Soybeans, peanuts, beans, peas, chickpeas, and lentils are some examples of legumes.

- **Seeds and nuts** are also staple foods in most meals. They are essential plant-based protein sources, omega-3 fatty acids, healthy fats, fiber, vitamin E, magnesium, calcium, iron, phosphorus, and selenium. Health benefits from plant-based diets are also linked to the consumption of seeds and nuts because they contain healthy omega-3 unsaturated fats and polyphenols with antioxidant abilities. Almonds, walnuts, hazelnuts, pecans, flaxseeds, hemp seeds, and chia seeds are some examples of nuts and seeds ranked healthiest.

- **Herbs and spices** are healthy and flavorful garnishes to a plant-based diet. They provide magnesium, folate, potassium, vitamins A, C, and K. They also aid your body in combating diseases. Thyme, ginger, cinnamon, and turmeric are some examples of herbs and spices that you can include in your plant-based diet.

This clears the misconception that a plant-based diet is boring. You also have to be creative with your meals by trying exotic plant-based ingredients. However, there are a few nutrients that plant ingredients cannot deliver in sufficient amounts, which we will discuss in the following section.

What Can't You Get from a Plant-Based Diet?

It is crucial to be aware of nutrients that are either difficult or impossible to obtain in adequate amounts from plant products. Such nutrients include vitamin B12, creatine, carnosine, vitamin D3 (cholecalciferol), heme iron, long-chain-omega-3 polyunsaturated fatty acids, and taurine. You will need to supplement these nutrients to your meals to obtain a balanced diet. Doing this helps you avoid malnutrition, a condition that causes frequent infections and reduced physical performance.

Vitamin B12

Vitamin B12 is a vital nutrient that is sufficiently obtained from animal-based products, such as meat, fish, eggs, and dairy products. It is also called cobalamin. Vitamin B12 is a nutrient that is required for the development of red blood cells. It is also responsible for maintaining normal brain and nerve function.

Despite nori seaweed being a suitable plant-based source of vitamin B12, it provides insufficient requirements. Weakness, fatigue, and impaired brain function characterize vitamin B12 deficiency. Vitamin B12 deficiency is also associated with neurological and psychiatric disorders (Grober et al., 2013). Babies of breastfeeding mothers suffering from vitamin B12 deficiency are also prone to developing neurological disorders. Too low vitamin B12 intake also contributes to heart and Alzheimer's diseases (Wang, 2002).

Vitamin B12 deficiency also leads to anemia due to insufficient or improper development of red blood cells. Therefore, when adhering to a plant-based diet, you do yourself a huge favor if you include supplements or eat vitamin B12-enriched food. Soy products, bread, enriched yeast extracts, and breakfast cereals are some examples of foods that are fortified with vitamin B12.

Long-Chain-Omega-3 Polyunsaturated Fatty Acids

Long-chain-omega-3 polyunsaturated fatty acids (n-3 LCPUFA) are essential fats needed for regulating cell membranes' fluidity. For this reason, n-3 LCPUFAs are crucial in maintaining the cell membrane functions, including cell division for growth and stopping the entrance of toxic substances in cells. Animal products are sources of n-3 LCPUFA, with fatty fish and egg yolks being the major providers. However, plant ingredients such as hemp seeds, chia seeds, flaxseeds, and walnuts contain omega-3 fats, which the body can transform into long-chain-omega-3 polyunsaturated fatty acids.

Creatine

Creatine is a molecule that is mainly reserved in your muscle and brain cells. It provides your muscle cells with the energy to increase endurance. Creatine is naturally found in animal tissues or products. However, it is not an essential diet requirement because your liver can produce it.

Contrastingly, Lukaszuk et al. (2002) found that people on a plant-based diet have reduced overall muscle creatine levels. Supplementing creatine significantly improves your physical and brain memory performance (Benton and Donohoe, 2010; Rae et al., 2003). Therefore, plant-based followers can take synthetic and non-animal-by-product creatine supplements.

Carnosine

Carnosine is a chemical that is also found in human and animal muscles and the brain. High levels of carnosine in your muscles improve physical performance while reducing muscle fatigue. Animal-based foods are the only sources of carnosine. Nevertheless, your body is able to synthesize carnosine from histidine and beta-alanine, which are amino acids. For this reason, carnosine is also disregarded as a vital diet requirement. Beta-alanine supplements improve your muscle mass and endurance by increasing the production of carnosine (Kern and Robinson, 2011).

Vitamin D3 (Cholecalciferol)

Vitamin D3, also known as cholecalciferol, is a fat-soluble secosteroid. It facilitates the absorption of phosphorus, magnesium, and calcium, all of which are essential in maintaining the strength of your bones. Egg yolks and fatty fish are the common rich sources of vitamin D3, in addition to increasing the levels of vitamin D in your blood. Cholecalciferol prevents rickets in children and the weakening of bones in adults. Lack of vitamin

D3 causes osteoporosis, which is the abnormal loss of bony tissue attributable to a lack of calcium. It also leads to osteomalacia, which is abnormal softening of bones as a result of phosphorus or calcium, or vitamin D deficiencies. Supplements of the nutrient include exposing your skin to the sun, which triggers the production of vitamin D. You can also get lichen-based vitamin D3 supplements.

Heme Iron

Heme iron describes a type of iron that is available only in animal flesh, such as red meat, fish, seafood, and poultry. Your body requires iron to produce hemoglobin, a vital protein in red blood cells that distributes oxygen to all body parts. Plant-based foods provide non-heme iron, the type that is absorbed at a relatively poor rate by the body, compared to heme-iron. Antinutrients, such as phytic acids in plant-based foods, limit non-heme iron absorption, but not heme iron. Therefore, plant-based food consumers are prone to iron deficiency, which causes anemia. Heme iron also facilitates the absorption of non-heme iron. Increase your intake of food rich in vitamin C, such as vegetables and fruits. Such foods promote the absorption of iron, thereby lowering the risks that are associated with iron deficiency.

Taurine

Taurine is an organic compound that is obtained naturally from fish, meat, and dairy products. It aids the growth of nerves in the brain, thus enhancing long-term memory (Shivaraj et al., 2012). The human body also produces taurine, though some people cannot produce it. The taurine deficiency is implicated in damaging neurons from the retina, a scenario that leads to loss of vision (Ripps and Shen, 2012). Intake of dietary taurine supplements would help to avoid such detrimental effects of insufficient taurine in the body.

Plant-Based Protein Products

Are you worried that you might suffer from protein deficiency by excluding any animal by-products from your diet? Fortunately, there are tons of plant ingredients that are rich in protein, which provide your body with essential and sufficient amino acids for bodybuilding and tissue repair. All you need to do is add plant-based protein ingredients when designing your meals. Major plant-based protein sources include

- **Whole grain:** Whole wheat is an unrefined grain that has been utilized to derive a meat substitute called seitan, which is packed with gluten protein. Whole grains such as wild and brown rice, oats, quinoa, amaranth, spelt, and teff are excellent sources of proteins.

- **Legumes:** Soybeans are highly packed with proteins. Fermenting soybeans produces a popular meat alternative called tempeh. Tofu is also a source of protein, and it is made from solidifying soy milk. The required daily intake of protein is approximately 46 grams for women to 56 grams for men. By simply eating 100 grams of premature soybeans called edamame, or tempeh and tofu, you add 10-19 grams of protein to your daily intake. You can also get another protein dose of 9 grams to 18 grams from 240 milliliters of legumes such as lentils, chickpeas, pinto beans, peanuts, and green peas. Edible seeds such as chia seeds, flax seeds, and hemp seeds are also excellent sources of proteins.

- **Nuts:** Almonds, pistachios, cashews, walnuts, hazelnuts, and peanuts are rich in protein which you can incorporate in meals. These nuts can add 4.5 grams to 9.5 grams to your daily requirements.

- **Fruits and vegetables:** All fruits and vegetables are plant-based protein sources. However, fruits such as guavas, jackfruit, avocado, apricot, kiwi, raspberries, and blackberries have more protein content, adding 2 grams to 4.2 grams to your daily requirements. Vegetables that are rich in protein include spinach, broccoli, asparagus, artichokes, potatoes, sweet potatoes, and Brussel sprouts.

- **Plant-based milk substitutes:** The production of plant-based milk substitutes continues to increase and is quite beneficial to those who subscribe to plant-based diets. Liquids from soybeans, flax seeds, hemp seeds, chia seeds, coconut, rice, almonds, oats, cashews, and peas have been used to produce plant-milk alternatives that you can add to your diet.

Plant-Based Doesn't Always Mean Healthy

Although plant-based foods have an excellent health and weight loss reputation, you need to watch out for significant pitfalls in the diet. Plant-based products also include refined sugars and grains, high salt and cholesterol, processed fat, and packaged convenience foods that are nutritionally deficient. Usually, some meat alternatives, such as meat-free burgers, are high in fat and salt. The American Heart Association states that high salt in meals raises your blood pressure, thereby increasing the risks of stroke and heart diseases. When you design your meals, emphasize organic food and supplements. In addition, you should practice healthy cooking methods like grilling, unlike using deep frying.

Benefits of a Plant-Based Diet

A plant-based diet includes ingredients with tons of medicinal properties that help present significant health benefits. Plant-based products are incredible immune boosters. This makes the diet even more appealing to consumers. Various studies revealed that this diet reduces the probabilities of diabetes, obesity, hyperlipidemia, heart disease, hypertension, high cholesterol, and some forms of cancer.

Scientists also suggest that following a diet that is centered on plants is a strategy for preventing meat-related health problems. It is also a significant drive for weight loss and management. Dietary fiber from plant sources is one of the critical elements that help in achieving these benefits. This section highlights the benefits that you will experience from following a plant-based diet.

Aids Weight-Loss

Designing your nutritionally balanced plant-based meals will definitely contribute to losing weight. A plant-based diet is an easy way to shed your excess weight because most plant foods are low in calories. Your body will compensate for low calories by burning stored fats to produce energy. One study showed that weight loss was attributed to switching from a meat-based diet to a plant-based diet (Tran et al., 2020).

A plant-based diet rich in fiber reduces belly fat. Several studies showed that ghrelin, a hormone that controls hunger in your body, is significantly reduced through high fiber intake (Hall et al., 2021). This is because your body digests fiber slowly, making you feel satiated for longer. This way, fiber reduces your intake of calories and facilitates weight loss. Consuming non-oil legumes, nuts, and seeds, such as lentils, black beans, almonds, and chickpeas, helps in weight loss. You can also add fruits and vegetables that are rich in fiber, such as avocados, bananas, and Brussel sprouts. Also, consider incorporating grains such as oats and wheat.

Carotenoids are chemicals that give fruits their color. These plant compounds also have antioxidant properties. Research reveals that this phytochemical also reduces insulin resistance. Increased intake of carotenoids was found to significantly lower body weight, while the decreased intake was associated with weight gain (Heather et al., 2010). Colorful fruits and vegetables such as mango, red bell pepper, carrots, sweet potato, and pumpkins are significant sources of carotenoids in the form of vitamin A.

Fruits and vegetables are also rich in another antioxidant called vitamin C. Research results showed that zinc intake from plant-based proteins reduces appetite, belly fat, and insulin resistance in obese patients (Khorsandi et al., 2019). You can increase your zinc intake by consuming cashew nuts, lentils, beans, and pumpkin seeds.

Lowers Risk of Diabetes

Turning to sustainable plant-based eating patterns is also an effective tool in preventing and managing diabetes. Studies revealed that adhering to a plant-based diet reduces your risk of type 2 diabetes by approximately 34% to 53% when compared to people who follow an animal-centered diet (Tina et al., 2018). This is because plant-centered foods are also able to maintain blood sugar levels.

Magnesium obtained from plant-based foods is essential in regulating blood glucose levels by reducing insulin resistance, which is a disorder where your body cells fail to absorb insulin. This hormone is vital for regulating blood glucose levels. Since the body cells cannot use the insulin, glucose concentrations in the blood increase to abnormal levels. High glucose levels impair weight loss because excess sugar is stored as fat in your body. Therefore, intake of plant-based foods rich in magnesium, such as soymilk, edamame, black beans, peanuts, cashews, and almonds, will help in reducing the risks of diabetes.

Reduces the Risk of Heart Disease

Adhering to a plant-based diet has always presented extraordinary interventions for preventing and reversing heart diseases. A study conducted by the American Heart Association found that the risk of heart disease is reduced by 52% when you eat meatless or minimal meat meals. Most plant products lower the risk of heart diseases by regulating blood cholesterol levels.

Animal food such as meat, eggs, poultry, and dairy products are high in solid or unhealthy saturated fat, which is bad because it tends to increase your low-density lipoprotein (LDL) cholesterol blood levels. Oxidized LDL cholesterol in the blood tends to reduce blood flow by forming fatty deposits in blood vessels. The formation of fatty deposits in arteries is known as atherosclerosis of coronary artery disease, and it increases the risks of stroke and heart attack. Plant products such as avocado, nuts, and olives have healthy unsaturated fat and low oil contents. Thus, substituting animal-saturated fat with plant-unsaturated fat decreases your cholesterol levels and risks of heart diseases.

Plant-based foods provide the body with nutrients that are natural interventions for decreasing your cholesterol levels. Eating tons of fruits and vegetables provides your body with antioxidants that prevent the oxidation of LDL cholesterol and the formation of plaques in blood vessels. This reduces the dangers of heart diseases. Herbs and spices like ginger, turmeric, cinnamon, mint, and garlic, are also plant-based ingredients that are jammed with antioxidants.

Plant chemicals such as anthocyanins, carotenoids, allicin, flavonoids, isoflavones, lignans, and phenolic acids in plant-based products also decrease blood pressure through antioxidation. Dietary intake of soluble fiber from plants also lowers cholesterol levels. Soluble fiber binds to cholesterol in the intestines. This prevents the absorption of cholesterol into the blood until it is eventually excreted.

Lowers Cognitive Decline

Cognitive status describes the functioning of the mind, including thinking, learning, reasoning, justifying, and remembering. Cognitive decline is when the mind slowly loses its functional efficacy. Some mental conditions that result from cognitive decline are amnesia, Alzheimer's disease, Lewy body dementia, and Huntington's disease.

Research emphasizes that cognitive decline can be strongly reduced by consuming more fruits and vegetables. Plant-centered meals significantly prolong the development of Alzheimer's disease and even reverse deficits in cognition (Malar and Devi 2014). This was attributed to antioxidants in plant products. (Xiang et al., 2017) highlighted that eating more fruits and vegetables would also reduce dementia by 20%.

High in Fiber

There are tons of plant-based foods with abundant fiber compared to animal products. Plants contain both soluble and insoluble forms of fiber. Soluble fiber helps to reduce blood glucose concentrations, cholesterol levels, diabetes, obesity, and heart diseases. Research has found that both soluble and insoluble fiber also reduce the development of cancerous cells in the digestive system.

Maintains the Digestive System

Dietary fiber is an essential nutrient that is classified as a carbohydrate. It is also known as bulk or roughage. Fiber also takes part in sustaining and increasing the growth of healthy bacteria in your gut. Healthy intestinal bacteria help in digestion by facilitating the absorption of nutrients like calcium. Insoluble fiber draws water and adds bulk to digested material, promoting the easy movement of digested material in the colon. This helps relieve constipation.

Lowers Risk of Cancer

Fiber is beneficial for reducing the development of certain cancers, especially those that are associated with the digestive system. A study by (Tantamango-Bartley et al., 2013) showed that people who ate meatless meals had significantly low chances of acquiring gastrointestinal cancer. The diets also reduced the probability of developing colorectal cancer, which was attributed to high fiber contents in plant-based meals.

Vitamins, minerals, and phytochemicals in plants boost your immune system. They reduce the odds of developing tumors in the stomach, rectum, esophagus, and pancreas. Some phytochemicals help to fight inflammation which can damage DNA and cause tumor growth. Antioxidants also reduce the damage to DNA that is caused by free radicals. They weaken the free radicals by neutralizing or scavenging them, thus decreasing the growth of the tumor.

It is Good for the Environment

Livestock rearing for meat and milk production poses negative impacts on the environment. Some of these changes contribute to climate change. It significantly occupies more land and pollutes water bodies. The practice of rearing livestock also accounts for 10 to 50 times greater global emissions of greenhouse gases than plant production (Poore and Nemecek, 2018).

Animal agriculture is also attributed to 5% of the global anthropogenic carbon dioxide emissions. This is because animal agriculture drives the clearing of large pieces of land by cutting down the trees that absorb carbon dioxide. This leads to high greenhouse gas levels. It also contributes to land degradation and soil erosion from cleared lands.

About 44% of emitted methane is also related to animal agriculture. Digestion in ruminant animals like cattle, goats, and sheep involves methane production, which is expelled through burping. Nitrogenous fertilizers for feed production are manufactured through burning fossil fuels that emit nitrous oxide. This also contributes 44% of emitted nitrous oxide, while agricultural plants only consume approximately 2% of the nitrogenous fertilizers.

It is estimated that animal agriculture will continue expanding to meet the increasing population demand. To reduce climate change, shifting to a plant-based diet reduces the environmental impacts that emanate from animal agriculture. Thus, this diet is regarded as sustainable and environmentally friendly.

Plant-Based Diets are Nutritionally for Everyone

Anyone can follow a plant-based diet and certainly get the essential nutrients that it provides. Your meals have to be nutritiously balanced. As the body transforms in different life stages, its nutritional requirements are also changed. The unique requirements are going to be discussed in the next section.

Infants and Pregnant Women

Infants and unborn babies require unique amounts of certain nutrients. Remember, weakness, fatigue, and impaired brain function characterize vitamin B12 deficiency. Infants and unborn babies demand supplements for vitamin B12 with omega-3 fatty acids to ensure proper development of the brain and nerves (Nemours Kidshealth, n.d.).

Kids also require more calcium content to support the development and maintenance of bone strength. Iron is also a key element in supporting the development of red blood cells. Breastfeeding and pregnant women also need vitamin B12, iron, and calcium supplements for their infants and fetuses.

Remember, fiber can reduce your appetite and limit the intake of calories. Fetuses and teens experience rapid growth and activity, which require more calories and proteins than adults. Thus, kids require less fiber than adults. Adding plant ingredients with more calories would help. Examples of such foods include soy products, whole grains, legumes, and nuts. Due to the fact that plant-based foods differ in nutrient contents, ensure that you feed your children with a variety of plant-based food options so that they acquire all nutrients.

2

PLANT-BASED DIETS AND WEIGHT LOSS

Plant-based diets are a great option if you intend to lose weight and maintain the desired weight for a lifetime. With this diet, you will finally be able to do away with the fad diets that always seemed to work in the first few weeks but would let you down in the long run. This chapter will provide you with a better perspective on how plant-based diets can help with weight loss. It includes a slight overview of what you should expect. This chapter is also laced with evidence from research that proves how plant-based diets can aid weight loss.

The Overview

Whether your goal is to lose weight, maintain your desired weight, or simply eat healthy, you can never go wrong with a plant-based diet. Losing weight can seem relatively straightforward in most cases, but keeping the weight off is the most challenging part. This can be pretty frustrating, especially if health reasons back the intention to lose weight. A plant-based diet that is followed consistently is a more natural and sustainable strategy for dealing with weight loss.

The calorie-counting moments that are associated with other diets that are designed to help you with weight loss can be pretty stressful. Did you know that stress causes weight gain, irrespective of the source? There are two reasons why stress causes weight gain. When you are stressed, your body releases two hormones—cortisol and adrenaline. The secretion of these hormones triggers a sudden increase of glucose in the bloodstream. This is meant to provide you with enough energy to deal with the "stressful" situation.

Once the stress is gone, the adrenaline and the blood sugar levels reduce to normal levels. That is when the negative impact of cortisol begins. This hormone increases your craving for sugar so that the blood sugar concentration rises again. The more you give in to such cravings, the more you increase your weight because the excess glucose in the blood is converted to fat for storage. This fat is what increases the body weight. This process repeats each time you experience the stress that is linked with diets that require you to count calories constantly. Just by adopting and sticking to a plant-based diet, you steer clear of that type of stress.

There is no need for calorie-counting when you are following a plant-based diet. This does not only save you from the stress involved but also from the stress-related weight gain.

Don't Expect the Weight-Loss to be Automatic

Please note that you don't automatically lose weight by eating a plant-based diet. Many other factors affect the rate at which you can lose weight. One of such factors is choosing the right meal plan and altering your lifestyle. If you are on a plant-based diet with an ineffective meal plan, the rate at which you lose weight is more likely to be slower. Here are some of the reasons why one can be on a plant-based diet and still be unable to lose weight:

- **Using too much cooking oil:** The plant-based diet on its own is very healthy, but how you prepare it matters much. For instance, when you use too much cooking oil in preparing your meals, you significantly increase the amount of calories that you consume in each meal. Plant-based foods are dense in nutrients but low in calorie content, while oils are low on nutrients but high in calorie concentrations. Just one tablespoon of oil has 14 grams of fat and 120 calories (Donahue, 2019). Besides having too many calories, oils do not take up much space in your digestive system. Therefore, you will not feel satiated, hence the need to consume even more food. The result of this is overeating. You can consider other meal preparation alternatives that do not include much oil. Salad dressings are a good example.

- **Eating out more often:** Meals prepared in restaurants often have more calorie content than those you prepare at home. This is because these meals are usually prepared with relatively larger amounts of oils, salt, and sugar. So, even if the meal is vegan, it still has more calories because of the preparation method adopted in restaurants. This might have insignificant effects if you eat out once in a blue moon. However, if you eat in restaurants more often and you are trying to lose weight on a plant-based diet, your chances of succeeding are limited.

- **Including less leafy vegetables in your plant-based diet:** A plant-based diet that is rich in leafy green vegetables like spinach and kale is more oriented toward weight loss. This is because these vegetables are nutrient-dense and have a low-calorie content. Moreover, these leafy vegetables are high in fiber, so they are digested at a much slower pace. This keeps you feeling satiated for longer, thereby reducing the urge to overeat.

The emphasis is not on Eliminating Carbohydrates.

Many weight-loss strategies that are out there emphasize eliminating or reducing carbohydrates while eating more proteins. While this might seem to be a viable approach, it is only feasible on a short-term basis. Such diets may cause cravings for sugars in the long run, leading to more frequent binging sessions. Additionally, losing weight is usually linked to better insulin sensitivity, which reduces the chances of getting type 2 diabetes. However, it has been noted that people who lose weight using diets that are high in protein forfeit this benefit. Their risk of suffering from type 2 diabetes is still high, even after losing weight (Physicians Committee for Responsible Medicine (PCRM), 2019). Other diets that limit protein intake but increase fat consumption, like the keto diet, are also associated with higher risks of diseases such as diabetes and heart disease.

On the contrary, plant-based diets are rich in carbohydrates, yet they are recommended for healthy weight loss. Ideally, three-quarters of your daily intake of calories should come from carbohydrates, particularly those sourced from vegetables, grains, beans, and fruits. Such carbohydrate intake is associated with lower risks of diabetes, obesity, and heart disease. That is why there is so much emphasis on eating whole foods or those that are minimally processed in plant-based diets.

The Link Between Weight-Loss and Plant-Based Diet

Plant-based foods have large amounts of fiber, making it easier for them to fill up your stomach without much calorie intake. This is one of the mechanisms of action that makes plant-based foods effective in aiding weight loss. To ensure weight loss, eat at least 40 milligrams of fiber every day (PCRM, 2019). This is relatively easy if you make vegetables, beans, and fruits the major components of your diet.

Cut down your consumption of fat-rich foods like cheese, eggs, meat, and oils. Did you know that one gram of fat that you get from fish, beef, or oil carries nine calories? This is quite a lot, and it is impossible to lose some pounds and keep them off with such eating patterns. Contrastingly, each gram of carbohydrates that you get from beans or potatoes only has four calories (PCRM, 2019). Eating these foods certainly gives hope for sustainable weight loss. In this section, much focus will be on how plant-centered foods promote weight loss.

Plant-Based Diets are Fiber-Rich

We can't talk about the weight loss that is dependent on eating plant-based diets without including the role of fiber. Even when one decides not to stick to a plant-based diet completely, adding some fiber to their diet will certainly improve the rate at which they lose weight—the weight-loss effects of including more fiber, even more, when you strictly follow a plant-based diet. The more fiber you eat, the more you feel fuller for longer. Including more fiber in your diet is a sustainable strategy for losing some pounds and keeping them off.

When you eat foods that are rich in dietary fiber, the bacteria that are resident in your digestive system begin to produce short-chain fatty acids. These fatty acids trigger the secretion of hormones that suppress appetite. This will reduce your meal frequency and the amount of food that you eat at one go.

In summary, fibers contribute to weight loss in three significant ways, which are

- Filling up the space in your gut, thereby reducing your food intake at an instance.

- Slowing down digestion so that you stay with the feeling of satiation for longer. This reduces your food intake over a period of time.

- Stimulating the release of appetite-suppressing hormones, thereby reducing your eagerness to eat.

Plant-Based Diets Create Calorie Deficit

Weight loss is a complicated phenomenon because there are many factors involved. One of such factors is that there should be a calorie deficit for weight loss to take place. Diets that are rich in plant-based foods make it easy for you to create that calorie deficit. This is because the same weight of a plant-based food already contains low amounts of calories compared to the same weight of animal-based food.

One study investigated the calorie intake of participants whose diets were either plant-based or animal-based keto diets (Hall et al., 2021). The participants were allowed to eat as much as they felt like, as long as they stuck to their diets. The results from the study showed that those who were on the keto diet ate 700 calories more than those who followed the plant-based diet. From these results, it could be extrapolated that plant-based diets make you feel fuller for longer, thereby reducing your overall food intake. This ultimately reduces the amount of calories that you take in through a diet that is plant-based.

Plant-Based Diets Enhance Insulin Sensitivity

Soon after eating your meal, glucose levels in the blood spike up. This is where the hormone called insulin comes in. Insulin reduces the blood glucose levels to normal, healthy levels by promoting its uptake by cells that will use the sugar for producing the energy that the body needs. Suppose the cells get enough glucose for the body's immediate energy needs; the excess glucose in the blood is converted to glycogen and stored in the liver and muscles. If sugar is still in excess in the blood, it is then converted to fat for storage. This last step promotes weight gain. The greater the fat storage, the more weight you gain.

If your body cells become resistant to insulin, this hormone will accumulate in the bloodstream. This scenario has two effects. First, the body cells won't be able to take up glucose, a state that increases the chances of the glucose being converted to fat. Second, higher insulin levels in the blood prevent fats from being broken down as an energy supply. Either way, the fat storage increases, which is more likely to cause weight gain.

Carbohydrates are often implicated as causes of insulin resistance because they are the ones that are converted to glucose that stock up in the bloodstream. This might be true for carbohydrates that come from sugary desserts, white bread, and cereals. On the contrary, evidence from research suggests that plant-based carbohydrates with fiber increase insulin sensitivity, thereby reducing cases of insulin resistance (McMacken and Shah, 2017). This helps to cut off unhealthy extra pounds and even keep them off.

Plant-Based Diets Improve Metabolism

One study revealed that plant-based diets can increase the rate and efficiency of metabolism (Kahleova et al., 2020). This can help to burn body fat, even without engaging in vigorous exercise. The study aimed to investigate whether a low-fat, vegan diet would improve metabolism and remarkably reduce weight.

To get better and more authentic results from the study, being overweight was one of the main aspects that guaranteed participation. The participants in the intervention group adopted a vegan diet for 16 weeks, while the control group continued with their everyday dietary habits. One of the significant aspects that were determined from the study was that the participants who followed the vegan diet lost weight. The researchers concluded that the weight loss was due to reduced insulin resistance and increased metabolism. More effective metabolism improves your body's ability to break down glucose and stored fats, enhancing weight loss.

Benefits of Losing Weight

We have extensively discussed how plant-based diets aid weight loss. However, it is also important to know why watching your weight is a crucial lifestyle habit. Apart from the need to fit in your beautiful outfits and other reasons, most people desire to lose weight for health reasons. Therefore, the benefits that we will address in this section are mainly health-related.

Better Cardiovascular Health

Individuals who are overweight have an increased chance of having fatty deposits in their arteries, a condition that is referred to as atherosclerosis. Such deposits reduce the available arterial diameter for blood to flow freely at a normal pressure. Instead, blood pressure increases to keep up with the body's needs for nutrients and oxygen. Such pressure can even damage the walls of the arteries. Moreover, being overweight is associated with an increase in low-density lipoprotein (LDL) cholesterol, also called 'bad cholesterol.' This type of cholesterol is labeled as 'bad' because it increases the chances of suffering from heart disease. Research shows that the risk of heart disease significantly reduces when you lose between 5% to 20% of your weight (Heger, 2020).

Reduces the Risk of Diabetes

When you are overweight, the adipose tissue in your body increases, adipose tissue is also known as body fat. It is commonly found coating internal organs, in the bone marrow, under the skin, as well as in breast tissue. As adipose tissue accumulates, it causes inflammation, in addition to interfering with the activity of insulin. This affects the role of insulin in regulating blood sugar levels, thereby increasing the risk of diabetes or worsening the condition if it is already there. This means when you lose weight, you automatically reduce your probability of getting diabetes. If you already have diabetes, losing weight better controls the condition. Interestingly, you don't have to lose many pounds to achieve the benefit; just a 5% reduction in your body weight can do the trick.

Reducing Severity of Sleep Apnea

Sleep apnea is a sleeping disorder that is common in individuals who are overweight. This is a condition whereby one experiences disrupted breathing while they are asleep. Sleep apnea can be caused by obstruction of the airways by the increased size of the neck due to weight gain. As a result, you cannot breathe properly, especially when you are sleeping. Losing weight is an effective prevention strategy for sleep apnea. However, if you already have the condition, losing weight won't completely cure the breathing discrepancy. It will improve the quality and quantity of your sleep, thereby reducing the severity of sleep apnea. You can make this possible by losing just 10% to 15% of your current weight (Heger 2020).

Cuts Down on the Risk of Stroke

Excess weight increases the risk of stroke because it can increase your blood pressure. Too high blood pressure strains the walls of your blood vessels, making them stiffer, apart from even increasing the chances of blood clots. The fact that weight loss normalizes blood pressure means that chances of stroking are equally cut down.

Decreased Pain in the Joints

Excess weight stresses your joints, causing them to become inflamed and even damaged. One study investigating the effect of losing weight in arthritis patients reported a significant reduction in joint pain upon losing 10% to 20% of body weight (National Institutes of Health, 2018). Weight loss reduces the pressure on the joints, thereby reducing the chances of them being damaged and painful.

Lower Risk of Specific Cancers

Approximately 5% of the cancers that affect males and 11% of those that affect women are attributed to being overweight. Some of the cancers that can easily affect people who are obese include kidney, endometrial, liver, breast, and pancreatic cancer. The link between cancers and weight gain remains unclear. However, researchers and scientists suggest that the fat that is found around internal organs, often known as visceral fat, is the cause of certain cancers. As such, the risk of suffering from such cancers can be reduced by weight-loss endeavors that reduce visceral fat.

Improved Mental Health

Losing weight is highly associated with better brain health. The results from one study revealed that women improved their ability to retain memory when they lost weight more than they did before their weight loss endeavors. These results showed that excess weight interferes with the proper functioning of the brain, especially cognitively. Being overweight is also linked to diseases that affect the brain, for example, Alzheimer's disease. Other studies also show that maintaining normal weight also aids better-concentrating acumen (Forer, 2011). Also, there has been an established link between excess weight and psychological issues such as depression, anxiety, and self-esteem.

3

THE FOODIE DOS AND DON'TS

This chapter will focus on clarifying the different types of plant-based diets that are available. We will also look at the different plant-based foods that you can include in your diet in order to lead a healthy lifestyle. The benefits of plant-based foods will be discussed in this chapter. Also included in this chapter are foods that you should avoid.

Currently, plant-based diets have become popular due to their numerous health and environmental benefits. It is important to note that when it comes to defining a plant-based diet, many explanations come to mind. Some people associate this diet with having plant-based foods only, without any meat or animal products. Others think that you can have plant foods in abundance, then limit meat and animal products. It should also be noted that others may think of a plant-based diet as one that contains plant-based foods and animal products such as eggs, cheese, and milk.

Lauren Manaker, an award-winning dietician, author, blogger, and nutrition expert, elucidated that your meals should be centered around plant-based foods. She said, "A plant-based diet emphasizes foods like fruits, vegetables, and beans, and limits foods like meats, dairy, and eggs." Manaker further explained that a plant-based diet could be made stricter, depending on your preferences. She suggested that "It may eliminate foods from animals or just limit intake, depending on the individual's interpretation." (Lawler, 2019).

Plant-Based Diets

There are also other diets that can be thought of as "plant-based diets." For instance, there are vegetarian and vegan, Mediterranean, and the Whole30 diets. The Whole30 diet is actually a diet that emphasizes animal proteins. However, it is feasible to qualify this diet as plant-based by strictly consuming plant-based foods instead of animal proteins.

A Vegetarian Diet

You may be drawn to this diet due to its potential health benefits. Others may follow the vegetarian diet for ethical or religious reasons. Vegetarian diets do away with beef and poultry. There are four main types of vegetarian diets, which are

- **The Lacto-vegetarian:** When you follow the Lacto-vegetarian diet, you will consume dairy products, but not fish, meat, poultry, and eggs.

- **The Lacto-ovo-vegetarian:** The Lacto-ovo-vegetarian diet allows you to have dairy and eggs, with the exclusion of fish, meat, and poultry.

- **The Ovo-vegetarian:** The Ovo-vegetarian diet is centered on egg consumption but excludes other animal products such as dairy, poultry, meat, and fish.

- **The Pescatarian:** This diet includes seafood, fish, honey, eggs, and dairy products. However, it excludes poultry and beef.

The primary focus of vegetarian diets is on vegetables, fruits, legumes, whole grains, seeds, and nuts. These foods provide a rich supply of micronutrients, fiber, and beneficial plant compounds called phytochemicals. Plant-based foods are lower in fat, calories, and protein in comparison with animal foods. The vegetarian diet is, therefore, associated with weight loss and the lowering of chronic disease risks.

The Vegan Diet

A vegan diet only consists of plant-based foods, including grains, nuts, fruits, vegetables, and plant product foods. Vegans do not eat any foods or products from animals, be it eggs, dairy, or honey. A healthy vegan diet should include five portions of vegetable and fruit varieties every day. Starchy carbohydrates such as rice, pasta, potatoes, and bread should be included as well. Where possible, you should opt for whole-grain starches (NHS Choices, 2018).

You could also consume some dairy alternatives like soy drinks and yogurts that are low in sugar and fat. As your protein source, consider having some pulses, beans, and other plant-based proteins. Small amounts of unsaturated spreads and oils are necessary when it comes to a healthy vegan diet. Also, include plenty of fluids in your vegan diet. If properly followed, a vegan diet is highly nutritious, aids weight loss, and decreases the risk of chronic diseases (Smith, 2020).

The Mediterranean Diet

The Mediterranean diet is a form of a plant-based diet that originates from the traditional cuisines of Italy, Greece, and other countries on the boundary of the Mediterranean Sea. The diet is characterized by vegetables, whole grains, fruits, legumes, seeds, nuts, herbs, and spices.

Olive oil is one of the most common sources of added fat. Olive oil is a good source of monounsaturated fat, which reduces the amounts of cholesterol and low-density lipoproteins, thereby reducing the risk of heart disease and aiding weight loss. Moreover, olive oil has a high smoke point of 374 F to 405 F. The smoke point of an oil refers to the temperature at which it breaks down, producing visible smoke. At this point, the oil releases harmful substances, mainly oxidative free radicals. These free radicals can cause degenerative diseases when they are consumed along with food. Since the smoke point of olive oil is higher than the average cooking temperature, the likelihood that it will decompose into harmful free radicals is relatively low. Therefore, olive oil is a safe alternative for cooking plant-based foods.

You can have seafood, fish, dairy, and poultry in moderate amounts in a Mediterranean diet. Fatty fish such as herring, mackerel, salmon, and sardines offer you a rich source of omega-3 fatty acids, which assist in combating inflammation. Omega-3 fatty acids also help to reduce triglycerides, thereby lessening the chances of blood clotting and the risk of heart failure and stroke. You can have meat and sweets only on certain occasions. This diet also allows you to have wine in moderation (Mayo Clinic Staff, 2019). Research revealed that the Mediterranean diet aids weight loss and contributes to preventing strokes, heart attacks, type 2 diabetes, and early death (Gunnars, 2018).

The Foods You Need

There are various types of foods that can be included in a plant-based diet. These include starchy and non-starchy vegetables, whole grains, legumes, fruits and berries, leafy greens, as well as herbs and spices. Each of the foods mentioned above has beneficial nutrients that they offer to enhance your health. Let's look at each of these in greater detail in this section.

Starchy and Non-Starchy Vegetables

As the name implies, starchy vegetables are rich in starch. Starch is a complex form of carbohydrate that can be broken down into glucose. In comparison with non-starchy vegetables, starchy vegetables contain more calories. Starchy vegetables are rich in antioxidants, minerals, and vitamins, making them a healthy choice to include in your diet. However, you should ensure to limit them to approximately a quarter of your plate. This is because starchy vegetables are high in carbohydrates, and they are more likely to spike your blood sugar. White potatoes, corn, sweet potatoes, beets, green peas, acorn squash, turnips, carrots, and butternut squash are examples of starchy vegetables.

Non-starchy vegetables contain higher fiber and low sugar when compared to starchy vegetables. These vegetables usually contain five grams of carbohydrates in each serving (webmd.com, 2020). A serving makes up a cup of leafy greens or half a cup of other frozen, fresh, or canned vegetables. You should fill half your plate with non-starchy vegetables. The list of non-starchy vegetables is endless, with some of them being eggplant, purple cabbage, black olives, asparagus, Brussels sprouts, white cabbage, celery, red peppers, summer squash, and tomatoes.

Starchy and Non-Starchy Vegetable Benefits

Both starchy and non-starchy vegetables provide you with a rich source of nutrients. It is essential that you include them in your diet. An interesting point to note is that the color of the vegetables represents the amounts of nutrients and antioxidants that they contain (webmd.com, 2020; McKinney, 2019). A rich antioxidant diet can decrease your risk of cancer and heart disease. It would be great to consume vegetables of different colors to exploit these vegetables' inherent antioxidant and nutrient properties.

- **Red:** Red vegetables, including tomatoes and beets, have antioxidants that reduce your risk of high cholesterol, blocked arteries, and high blood pressure. The red compounds improve brain function and aid in protection against cancer.

- **Purple and blue:** The purple and blue vegetables, such as purple cabbage and eggplant, have antioxidants that assist in preventing stroke, cancer, and heart disease. They are also responsible for healthy aging as well as a healthy memory. Furthermore, they improve digestion and urinary tract health.

- **Orange and yellow:** Inclusive of these types of vegetables are pumpkins, carrots, and sweet potatoes. Orange and yellow vegetables are rich in nutrients and antioxidants that enhance eye health, prevent heart disease, maintain healthy skin, assist in building strong bones, and boost the immune system.

- **Green:** Green vegetables such as spinach and broccoli

help in protecting your eyes from macular degeneration, which is the deterioration of the retina that can lead to impairment of vision (webmd.com, 2019). Macular degeneration exists in two types, which are dry and wet macular degeneration. Dry macular degeneration involves the direct deterioration of the retina, while wet macular degeneration describes the condition where leaky blood vessels start to grow under the retina. Green vegetables also protect you from bad cholesterol and cancer. The antioxidants in green vegetables improve your immune system and assist in controlling digestion. Green vegetables are also vital for pregnant women because they have folic acid, which helps to prevent birth defects.

- **White:** Onions and cauliflower are examples of white vegetables that enhance your immune system function. White vegetables reduce bad cholesterol and enhance normal blood pressure. They also have nutrients that protect against some types of cancer.

Some starchy vegetables such as sweet potatoes, green plantains, peas, beans, and lentils contain resistant starches. This starch type is indigestible in the small intestines, so it does not elevate your glucose. The large intestine houses resistant starch fermentation. Your gut bacteria are enhanced as the resistant starch is fermented. Resistant starch increases your satiety, and this is important in glycemic regulation. Your cholesterol is decreased, constipation is prevented, and your risk of colon cancer is lowered by consuming plant-based foods that contain resistant starches.

Starchy vegetables such as chickpeas, lentils, and beans are rich in protein, apart from the starch that they contain. These vegetables are good plant-based protein sources, which consist of approximately nine grams of protein in 70 to 90 grams (Coyle, 2018). The amount of protein in these vegetables makes them incredible alternatives for meat in vegan and vegetarian dishes. The protein content of beans, chickpeas, and lentils promotes satiety, thereby keeping your weight and appetite in check. Preservation of muscle mass and strength are the other beneficial characteristics of these vegetables.

It is recommended to consume your vegetables while they are still fresh or as frozen whole vegetables. You could also have them juiced or canned, but the fresh or frozen options are better. Bear in mind that the preparation and cooking procedures affect the nutritional quality of vegetables. Consider cooking methods such as steaming, boiling, and baking for your vegetables and avoid unhealthy condiments to curb additional calories, fat, and salt. Try to limit your consumption of unhealthy, processed, and fried vegetables. Foods that are prepared this way have compromised nutritional value. Moreover, they might contain oxidative free radicals, especially if the frying is done using unhealthy oils with low smoking temperatures. Regularly consume starchy and non-starchy vegetables in order to enhance your nutrient and vitamin intake.

Whole Grains

Whole grains are crucial to a healthy diet, and they have been seen to be beneficial to human health in numerous ways. Naturally, they are rich in fiber, which makes you feel full and satiated, thereby helping you to sustain a healthy body weight. Furthermore, whole grains are associated with a reduced risk of diabetes, heart disease, and certain cancers. The Dietary Guidelines for Americans recommend that half of all the grains you eat should be whole grains (Mayo Clinic Staff, 2017).

Apart from whole grains, there are also refined grains and enriched grains. Refined grains are those that have had their germ, bran, or endosperm removed with the aim of creating a finer texture. Enriched grains are those that have some nutrients added to them. The added nutrients may naturally belong to the particular grain that is being enriched. Both refined and enriched grains have most of their nutrients removed, so they are not as healthy as whole grains. In this section, we will discuss more on whole grains.

Whole grains are seeds that come from grasses that are cultivated for food. They are rich sources of manganese, magnesium, iron, selenium, iron, dietary fiber, and vitamins (Raman, 2018). They range from huge kernels of corn to tiny quinoa seeds. Other examples of whole grains include rice, bulgur, barley, oatmeal, millet. It is of utmost importance to check the nutritional content list or product label to ensure that your food really contains whole grains. Sometimes, the manufacturers may add some products that appear to be whole grains. Therefore, be cautious and ensure that you check the product label beforehand.

Some Tips for You to Enjoy Whole Grains

While whole grains are beneficial to your health, it may not be easy for you to consume them at the frequency that helps you to sequester the benefits. In this section, we will have more insight into how you can include whole grains in your diet.

- For additional bulkiness, you could add whole-grain bread crumbs to your ground meat or poultry.

- Instead of having white rice, have quinoa, barley, bulgar, or rice.

- Include barley or wild rice in stews, soups, and salads.

- When making sandwiches, try to use whole-grain rolls or bread.

- Fill your breakfasts with whole-grain cereals such as whole-wheat bran flakes.

Legumes

A healthy plant-based diet will consist of legumes. Legumes are the fruits or seeds that grow in pods. Examples of legumes include peanuts, soybeans, fresh beans or peas, and pulses. Any type of legume that contains dried seeds inside the pod is called pulses. Legumes provide you with protein, iron, fiber, zinc, folate, magnesium, phosphorus, and selenium.

The consumption of legumes improves heart health by lowering bad cholesterol. When your body has low levels of bad cholesterol, it is highly unlikely that heart disease will result. Consuming legumes helps to curb appetite, thereby managing weight. Eating legumes is linked to a reduction in waist circumference. These legumes also aid in the regulation of blood sugars.

Please note that there are considerations that you should take in order to obtain maximum absorption of some of the nutrients available in legumes. For instance, zinc absorption can be improved by cooking, soaking, sprouting, or fermenting legumes. In addition to the aforementioned nutritional properties of legumes, soybeans and soy products also have omega-3 fatty acids and vitamin E. In products such as tofu and fortified soy beverage, you can obtain calcium, which improves your bone health.

Fruits and Berries

Fruits and berries provide you with a vast amount of nutrition. There is a famous saying which says, "An apple a day keeps the doctor away," which shows how important it is to consume fruits. Individual fruits and berries have unique nutrients, as well as benefits that they offer to your body. Consuming fruits helps you to decrease blood pressure and lower the risk of heart disease, stroke, some cancers, as well as digestive and eye problems. Another important aspect is that fruits positively impact your blood sugar, thereby controlling your appetite and subsequently aiding weight loss. Examples of fruits to include in your plant-based diet are apples, mangoes, avocados, lychees, and pineapples.

Apples have a rich supply of soluble and insoluble fibers like pectin, cellulose, and hemicellulose. These are beneficial in maintaining your blood sugar, heart, and gut health and aiding digestion. Apples also provide you with plant polyphenols and vitamin C, which help in combating diseases. Regular consumption of apples reduces your risk of stroke, heart disease, cancer, and obesity (Davidson, 2021).

Mangoes provide you with numerous plant phenols that provide you with anti-inflammatory and antioxidant characteristics. They also offer a great source of folate, potassium, fiber, together with vitamins A, C, B6, E, and K. Mangoes help to protect you from heart disease, type 2 diabetes, as well as some types of cancer. They also contain fiber, which is good for supporting bowel movements and helps with digestion.

Berries are fruits that contain seeds, and they result from a single ovary of an individual flower (Leafyplace.com, 2019). It is important to note that the botanical meaning of berries qualifies fruits such as grapes, cucumbers, and even bananas as berries. However, in the culinary world, berries include strawberries, cranberries, and raspberries. The benefits of these delicious and highly nutritious berries include their antioxidant properties, regulation of blood sugar, provision of numerous nutrients, and assistance in fighting inflammation (Spritzler, 2016).

Leafy Greens

Leafy greens contain nutrients such as fiber, vitamins B, C, and K, folate, beta carotene, magnesium, potassium, calcium, and iron. These vegetables are low in calories, and each of them offers an exceptional mixture of nutrients. That is why it is important to have a variety of vegetables in your plant-based diet. Leafy greens are rich in antioxidants, for example, polyphenols and carotenoids. Antioxidants are advantageous because they decrease the risk of some cancers, cardiovascular diseases, stroke, macular degeneration, depression, and diabetes.

The other benefits of leafy greens are improved sleep quality, lung function, and improvements in asthma symptoms. Having leafy, fibrous vegetables decreases the risk of metabolic syndrome. Polyphenols are also helpful with brain health.

Leafy greens have a compound called oxalate, which is an anti-nutrient. Oxalates may interfere with calcium absorption. Some leafy greens have high amounts of oxalate, while others have low ones. If you are a vegan, consuming leafy greens low in oxalate is recommended to increase calcium absorption and subsequently improve your bone health.

For the high oxalate leafy greens, be sure to boil them first. Afterward, discard the water. This allows you to reduce the oxalate concentration in the leafy greens, thereby promoting calcium absorption. Leafy greens that are low in oxalate include kale, turnip greens, broccoli, and collard greens. Those that are high in oxalate include beet greens, spinach, endive, and Swiss chard.

If you can, consuming raw leafy greens can be more beneficial. It has been known that some nutrient content may be lost due to cooking or freezing, although much of the nutritional value is preserved. As mentioned above, boiling or cooking some greens is helpful when it comes to making some nutrients readily available for absorption.

Herbs and Spices

Herbs and spices can enhance any plant-based diet. They provide you with good flavors, in addition to the health benefits that they offer. When it comes to weight management, herbs and spices are advantageous in that they are used in small amounts, so they will not present weight gain challenges to your diet.

Herbs and spices can provide you with nutrients such as magnesium, fiber, vitamins C and K, folate, iron, potassium, and calcium. Spices contain numerous antioxidants and may help in fighting cancer. Insulin regulation is another advantage of consuming spices. Examples of herbs that you can consume include basil, rosemary, oregano, mint, and sage.

The Foods You Don't Need

Apart from the beneficial foods that we discussed earlier, there are also other foods that adversely affect your health. It is essential to avoid these types of foods so that you avoid unnecessary health complications. Some of the foods that you should avoid include processed foods, unsweetened plant-based milk and beverages, sweeteners, and animal products. Vegan alternatives such as vegan cheeses and ice cream or meat alternatives should be avoided at all costs. Although all these may appear to be great alternative options, it should be noted that they are not healthy. Consuming them will lead to the development of disease and may result in premature death. Let's discuss each of these in more detail in this section.

Processed Foods

If a particular food has been changed from its natural state, during preparation, the food is defined as processed. It can be as simple as freezing, baking, canning, and drying (NHS Choices, 2019). Although sometimes it can be beneficial to process food, most food processing has adverse effects on your health. This is because, during processing, most of the nutrients are lost. Examples of processed foods are breakfast cereals, canned vegetables, plant-based meats, and savory snacks such as chips, cookies, and pies.

The American Academy of Nutrition and Dietetics suggests that there is a range for processed food, from minimally to mostly processed ones. Health risks increase as we move towards the most processed foods on the scale. Whenever possible, it is crucial to avoid heavily processed foods.

Processed foods become less healthy when various ingredients, including sugar, salt, and fat, are added. Adding these ingredients is done to create a more flavorful food, extend shelf life, and sometimes contribute to the structure of the food. Consuming processed foods will result in you having more amounts of sugar or salt above the recommended values. The consumption of processed foods also tends to increase your calorie intake, thereby leading you to put on more weight and be exposed to weight-gain-related diseases.

Unsweetened Plant-Based Milk and Beverages

Although many plant-based kinds of milk are enriched with many nutrients, not all of them are. Many of them do not contain vital nutrients such as potassium, protein, and vitamin D (MacKeen, 2021). A link has been established in young children between rickets and soy beverages, kwashiorkor, and rice beverage, with metabolic alkalosis being linked to almond-based drinks (Vitoria, 2017). From this information, it is clear that you should stay away from unsweetened plant-based milk and beverages.

Sweeteners

Artificial sweeteners come in handy for food manufactures because they are used as additives in processed foods. These are offered to people as a solution for weight loss. However, it is essential for you to understand the adverse effects associated with consuming these sweeteners. To begin with, artificial sweeteners are chemicals that have been made in the laboratory, which serve no benefit or function to the human body (Kay, 2018). These sweeteners promote food cravings, thereby leading to weight gain.

Artificial sweeteners are also responsible for harming gut bacteria, which then leads to skin and digestive issues. The overall effect is the disruption of the function of gut bacteria, which leads to a weakened immune system. There are natural sweeteners such as Stevia. Although this is a natural product, there are inherent issues of concern associated with it. Stevia may have adverse effects on your reproductive system, kidneys, and cardiovascular system (McDermott, 2018). Therefore, try to avoid the consumption of sweeteners.

Animal Products

Cow's milk has approximately three times the amount of protein and an additional 50% fat as opposed to human milk (peta.org, 2010). Consuming animal products is associated with cancer, heart disease, arthritis, diabetes, and osteoporosis. In

South Africa, research revealed no incidence of rheumatoid arthritis in a community where the people did not consume dairy products or meat (peta.org, 2010). This is evident that cutting down or not having meat and animal products promotes good health.

In Britain, people have become motivated to cut down on their meat consumption, with 49% having an appreciation that consuming too much meat might adversely affect their health (independent.co.uk, 2017). Research revealed that having animal products makes them more exposed to lactose, cholesterol, saturated fat, harmful microorganisms, and estrogens while doing away with complex carbohydrates, fiber, and antioxidants, together with other vital components necessary for health (Barnard and Leroy, 2020). The consumption of animal products will then lead to increased risks of diabetes, cardiovascular disease, cancer, obesity, and other ailments. It is, therefore, crucial to stick to plant-based diets for the promotion of good health.

Vegan Alternatives

In the United States, people are opting for plant-based meats for various reasons, including health. Plant-based meat can provide you with nutrients, but it is important to explore the nutritional shortcomings that come with these vegan alternatives. Vegan alternatives may contain fillers as well as added sodium (Richards, 2021). They may also contain high levels of saturated fats. Another characteristic of plant-based meats is that they may have less zinc and other minerals, as opposed to regular meat. These reduced amounts of zinc and the high levels of saturated fats will have a negative impact on your health.

4

THE PLANT-BASED TIPS

C hanging to a plant-based lifestyle may seem socially and emotionally intimidating, especially when you are transitioning from a full-fledged meat diet. The journey may seem short or long, but you don't need to feel the pressure for a quick switch. Instead, have patience and embrace the process. In this section, our goal is to highlight a few tips on making your transition and adjustment to a plant-based lifestyle easier.

Prepare Yourself

Making the plant-based diet your main diet requires you to prepare yourself, especially if it's your first time. Your mindset needs to be oriented toward your new diet. Mind you, you will be tempted to eat foods that are not part of the plant-based diet here and there, but you still have to remain focused. Here are three main ideas that will keep you firm as you pursue your dream diet.

Be Goal-Oriented

Knowing the reason(s) why you are turning to a plant-based diet is important because it enhances your commitment. Your goal is losing weight and maintaining it at desired levels through plant-based diets. Write your goal on paper and put it where you can frequently and easily see it as a reminder that keeps you going. For instance, you can stick the note to your dressing mirror, computer screen, or fridge. You could also set a daily reminder on your phone along with motivational messages like, "I can do it!"

Change Your Mindset

An effective strategy would be approaching the process with a positive and enduring mindset. Think of this journey as an adventure to new and exciting discoveries of food, flavor, and health benefits. Consider it as an advance to a plant-based diet rather than some form of deprivation.

Plan Your Approach

Planning helps you to clarify your approach throughout the transition. Choose a step-by-step approach that will gradually guide you in the process of adopting the plant-based diet. First, break your long-term goal into smaller goals that will lead you to be a seasoned and faithful follower of the plant-centered diet. For instance, if your primary goal is losing weight, your smaller goals could be reducing your calorie intake, adjusting to exercising, and getting rid of your unhealthy cravings. Basically, the smaller goals together form the roadmap that will see you adopting the plant-based diet with increased ease.

Proceed to outline your short-term goals and separate them into steps that you can manage and follow through. Your first goals should be the easiest but gradually lead to the difficult ones. This helps you to build up resilience as you go and avoid quitting. Schedule meals that correspond to each goal on your list. Clearly write them down so that you are able to control what you eat. You can also tick the mini-goals that you have achieved to keep track of your progress at every stage in the transition. This also keeps you motivated. You should also make a grocery list that complements your plan. This helps to stock up on what you need, save money, and control your meals.

Go Meatless

When you are ready to start, you have to take other practical steps that assist you in achieving your goal of starting to eat a plant-based diet. One of the most important aspects of a plant-based diet is reducing meat consumption to finally eliminate it. In this section, we will explore aspects that you should consider as you go 'meatless.'

Make the Transition Slow

After planning, your next stage would be implementing, which can be pretty daunting. It can be overwhelming to suddenly give up all your meat-based ingredients at once. Instead, keep it simple, start with one goal, focus on it, and follow the process. For instance, gradually remove one ingredient at a time so that your taste buds can adjust to plant-based alternatives. The first alteration to your diet should be easy. We have compiled suggestions for your slow transition from other diets that involve animal products to a plant-oriented diet.

Adjust Your Plant-Based Portions

It's not only important to eliminate meat but to increase your plant ingredients, too. Start by including plant-based ingredients in every meat meal. Simply move on to adjusting the meat to vegetable ratio in your meals—dish larger portions of plant-based foods than meat. Before long, you will be able to incorporate meat as a garnish to your plant-based ingredients, rather than it being the basis. Adding plant-based ingredients would provide you with the nutrients your body needs and add the fiber that helps you lose weight.

Reduce Your Meat Consumption

Your next step would be substituting at least one animal-based meal with a meatless meal per week. Incorporating the popular Meatless Mondays slogan would help reduce your meat intake by coupling it with some fun. As you adjust, expand to three more meatless meals until you are more comfortable to have one meat-based meal per week.

Your next stage would be making a daily goal of committing to one meatless meal. Begin with plant-based breakfasts and move to plant-based lunches and dinners. During this period, concentrate on trying new ingredients and recipes that are plant-based. Explore plant-based meat substitutes. For instance, if you enjoy chicken stew, replace the meat with soy chunks, tempeh, seitan, or mushrooms. Also, gradually adopt your favorite veggie meals to swap with meat dishes. This will help you to gently familiarize yourself with the new diet.

Eliminate Meat From Your Diet

Once you are used to spending a whole day or week without meat, it becomes easy to eliminate meat from your diet. To do this, start by removing meat types, for example, having four-legged animal meat once a week and gradually moving toward a month until you eventually chuck it out. You can also follow the same process for poultry and seafood. Following this process will help you accommodate the changes, commit, and eventually eliminate meat from your diet without feeling like you are depriving yourself of some goodies.

Substitute Animal-Based Milk and Yogurt

Eliminating meat makes the rest of the animal products easier to give up, such as milk. Animal-based milk is directly substituted by a wide range of plant-based milk that is made from almond, chia, coconut, rice, soy, hemp, pea, oat, or peanut. You can either buy ready-made plant-based milk or follow easy homemade recipes to make milk from plant-sourced ingredients. For instance, to make your homemade milk, you soak almonds or cashews in water overnight before draining, rinsing, and blending them with water until they are smooth. You can then collect the milk by filtering it through a cheesecloth or strainer.

As time progresses, replacing yogurt also becomes effortless. You can easily produce yogurt from cashews, almonds, soybeans, coconuts, and oats on your own. There is also an array of yogurt options on the market.

Displace Animal-Based Cheese and Cream

Cheese is one of the ingredients that are embraced in animal-based diets. You can replace it with store-bought non-dairy cheese options like Mozzarella, Gouda, cheddar, cream cheese, and parmesan. You can also consider learning how to prepare homemade cheese (Piatt, 2017). Spend time to experiment on homemade plant-based sauces and creams using tofu or cashews.

Avocado is tasty, thick, and creamy, making it an excellent replacement for dairy-based sour cream, mayonnaise, pudding, and spreads. Hummus is another fantastic alternative to replace plant-based dips and spreads. It can be homemade with mashed chickpeas, salt, tahini, garlic, and lemon juice. Adjust to these alternatives for a short period and cut out dairy products in the long run.

Remove Eggs

You might be wondering about what can replace eggs in baking. Flax eggs, banana, chia eggs, soft tofu, aquafaba, and applesauce are easy replacements for eggs. Do this gradually until you finally remove eggs to achieve your plant-based diet.

It's More Than Going 'Meatless'

A plant-based diet is more than just going meatless. There are many other aspects that make it successful and effective. We will discuss some of such elements in this section.

Aim for Whole Foods

As the change from an animal-based diet to a plant-based one becomes habitual, add another goal to convert to a whole-food plant-based diet. Carbohydrates don't necessarily promote weight gain on their own; what you combine with them is what matters. Combining ingredients such as butter, oil, and sugars with foods rich in carbohydrate foods contributes to weight gain and heart disease. Such unhealthy ingredients are common in processed and refined plant-based products that are also nutritionally deficient in fiber, minerals, and calories.

Indulge in whole plant-based ingredients rather than highly processed or refined plant-based food. Allow yourself to enjoy new tastes and eliminate unhealthy junk food. Incorporate high-quality carbohydrates of the right quantity from whole grains to your balanced diet. Whole grains, such as rice, quinoa, farro, rolled oats, barley, and amaranth, are healthy sources of carbohydrates.

Know Your Nutrients

Remember that vitamin B12 is impossible to obtain from plant sources. There are also other nutrients that are insufficiently absorbed from plant ingredients. However, aim for a variety of colorful and whole plant-oriented ingredients so that you can satisfy all your nutritional requirements. A weight-loss diet also emphasizes a colorful plate of plant ingredients. This section stresses on nutrients that you need to consider on a plant-centered diet.

Vitamin B12

Plant products provide the body with all other nutrients except for vitamin B12. It is recommended to complement your plant-oriented diet with vitamin B12 supplements. Eat food that has been enriched with vitamin B12 like nutritional yeast, cereals, and bread. You have to take enough supplements to meet your optimal daily requirement, which is 2.4 micrograms. Be sure not to overdose to levels that are deemed toxic.

Vitamin D

Remember, vitamin D3 is commonly obtained from egg yolks and fatty fish. Supplements of the nutrient include exposing your skin to the sun, which triggers the production of vitamin D. However, human lives involve being indoors most of the time and wearing clothes at work, school, or home. You could also be living in a region where you don't get enough sun rays. This means that the ability of the human body to absorb enough sunlight is limited. Therefore, supplementing vitamin D becomes essential.

There are plant-based vitamin D supplements that have been derived from mushrooms or algae. Plant-based milk has also been enriched with about 84 IU per 100 grams of vitamin D (U.S. Food and Drug Administration, 2018). You can also get lichen-based vitamin D3 (cholecalciferol) supplements. To test if you are getting enough vitamin D, get a blood test that measures the concentration of 25-Hydroxy Vitamin D in your serum.

A healthy and optimal level for vitamin D should be above 30 nanograms per milliliter but below 50 nanograms per milliliter (Institute of Medicine, Food and Nutrition Board, 2010). According to the Endocrine Society, adults need to supplement 37.5 to 50 micrograms of vitamin D per day. They also state that adolescents and kids require at least 25 micrograms of vitamin D per day (Holick et al., 2011).

Protein

The required daily intake of protein is approximately 46 grams for women and 56 grams for men. Children of 9 to 13 years should meet 34 grams, 4 to 8 years require 19 grams, and 2 to 3 years need 13 grams of protein per day. Eating a wide range of whole plant-based food in a balanced diet will help you satisfy your protein requirements.

Ensure that plant-based protein foods are included in most of your meals. Incorporating 100 grams of legumes such as lentils, soy products, chickpea, chia seeds, pinto beans, and peanuts provides about 3 to 19 grams of protein. Eating 25 grams of nuts, such as almonds, pistachios, cashews, walnuts, hazelnuts, and peanuts, can add 4.5 to 9.5 grams of proteins to your meals.

All fruits are plant-based sources of approximately 1 gram to 4.2 grams of protein. Fruit sources of higher protein content include jackfruit, avocado, blackberries, kiwi, raspberries, and apricots. Better sources of protein from vegetables are broccoli, mushrooms, and kale which contain about 4 grams of protein. Whole grains, such as quinoa, teff, wild rice, and oats, provide about 4 to 13 grams of protein. Plant-based dairy alternatives, such as unsweetened soy milk, contain about 7 grams, while almond milk provides approximately 1 gram of protein per cup (Krans, 2020).

Omega-3 Fatty Acids

Plant ingredients, such as seaweeds, are direct sources of long-chain omega-3 fatty acids: Docosahexaenoic acid (DHA) and Eicosapentaenoic acid (EPA). However, these amounts are inadequate. As an alternative, the human body requires omega-6 fatty acid, also called linoleic acid (LA), an omega-3 fatty acid, also known as alpha-linolenic acid (ALA), to derive EPA and convert EPA to DHA. Walnuts, soybeans, flax, hemp, and chia seeds are excellent ALA omega-3 fatty acids sources.

However, the human body doesn't derive sufficient requirements of DHA and EPA from ALA. Therefore, it is recommended to consider supplementing your plant-based diet with DHA and EPA derived from algae. The amount of DHA and EPA that you should take per day has not been successfully recommended yet as research is still in progress. However, these studies still give insights that suggest a DHA daily dose of 300 milligrams for adults (Vegan Health and Evidence-Based Nutrient Recommendations, n.d.).

Zinc

Another essential nutrient to consider is zinc. The human body depends on zinc for various functions, such as stimulating enzymes, nerves, and gene regulation. This micronutrient also aids the immune system in combating systemic inflammation.

Zinc is abundantly attained from nuts, legumes, seeds, and grains.

It is important to note that plant-based foods also contain phytates, which are antinutrient phytochemicals. Phytates chelate zinc ions, thereby making them unavailable for absorption in the body. This may result in zinc deficiency. To reduce the effects of phytates, use food preparation methods that lower the amounts of phytates in food. For example, roasting nuts or soaking beans and grains reduce their phytate content. You can also consume soy-derived food such as tempeh and tofu. If you are not getting enough zinc, you can take a daily supplement of 11 micrograms for men and 8 grams for women.

Iron

As we highlighted earlier, the body poorly absorbs non-heme iron from plants than heme iron from animal products. Simply eat a variety of healthy plant-based foods, such as lentils, quinoa, soybeans, rice, cashews, pumpkin seeds, collard greens, and prune juice. To increase the absorption of non-heme iron from plants, consider combining a plant-based non-heme iron food like brown rice or potatoes with plant-based vitamin A or C sources, such as carrots, broccoli, green, and red peppers.

Calcium

Calcium is essential in building and maintaining the strength of your bones. The required daily intake of calcium is 1000 to 1200 milligrams for adults. Many plant-based foods provide calcium, especially soybeans and soy-derived products, like tofu, natto, and tempeh. You can get 350 milligrams of calcium phosphate from 100 grams of tofu. Legumes, such as beans, lentils, and peas, are also good sources of calcium. Sesame, flax, and chia seeds can provide about 13% of the recommended dietary intake (RDI) per 20 to 25 grams.

Nuts, such as almonds, walnuts, and Brazil nuts, can provide 2 to 10% of the RDI to balance your nutrients. Grains, such as teff, brown rice, oats, and amaranth, provide 12% to 15% of the RDI. Eating a variety of vegetables, such as mustard, turnip, and spinach supply 8 to 14% of the RDI. Oranges, raspberries, figs, and blackberries provide 2% to 7% of the RDI. A cup of fortified plant-based milk provides approximately 283 to 451 milligrams of calcium.

Vitamin K2

Vitamin K exists in two forms, which are vitamin K1 and K2. Vitamin K1 can be easily obtained from green leafy vegetables. However, vitamin K2 is abundantly available in animal-sourced foods and fermented plant products. Fermented soybeans produce natto and miso dishes, which contain vitamin K2. However, you won't know if you are taking adequate amounts because fermenting doesn't give the amount of vitamin K2 in the product. Thus, you should consider supplementing 10 to 25 micrograms of vitamin K2, as suggested by Dr. Andrew Weil (Weil, 2011).

Selenium

Selenium is an essential nutrient necessary for protecting the structure and function of nerve cells. The deficiency of selenium causes neurodegeneration, which is a gradual degeneration and death of nerve cells. A few plant-based foods contain selenium. These include Brazil nuts, brown rice, sunflower seeds, baked beans, oatmeal, spinach, lentils, cashews, mushrooms, and bananas. There are also plant-based selenium fortified foods, which include whole-wheat bread and whole-grain cereal. The recommended daily intake of selenium is 55 micrograms for individuals over 14 years, 40 micrograms for 9- to 13-year-olds, 30 micrograms for 4- to 8-year-olds, 20 micrograms for seven months- to 3-year-olds, and 15 micrograms for those below six months (Bendich, 2001). Lactating or pregnant women require an adequate selenium daily intake of 60 micrograms.

Iodine

Iodine is essential because the human body utilizes it to synthesize thyroid hormones. Apart from the seaweed, plant foods are poor sources of iodine. However, adequate iodine can be obtained from fortified plant-based milk.

Limit the Oil or Cut it out Completely!

Plant-based oils are absolutely a better option for cooking than butter. Replace unhealthy saturated fats with less harmful plant-based oils. However, plant-based oils still have an impact on arteries, which could eventually increase your risk of heart disease. Oils also tend to add more calories to your food, thus contributing to weight gain. Start by limiting the amount of oil you use and gradually adjust to replacing it with liquids, such as water, fruit juice, and vinegar. Unsweetened applesauce, mashed bananas, and pears are great substitutes for oil when baking. Continue accommodating the changes until you can eliminate the oils.

More Tips

When you are able to incorporate the ideas that we discussed earlier, you will undoubtedly become a full-fledged plant-based dieter. This section recommends more tips to make the process less daunting and improve your weight-loss goals through plant-based diets.

Never Skip a Meal

A plant-based meal goes against starving yourself. Instead, balance the amount of calories and nutrients in your meals.

Skipping meals deprives your body of essential nutrients and energy. Unfortunately, skipping meals will draw you to unhealthy snacking because of starvation. Snacking on unhealthy food contributes to gaining weight. Skipping meals will also result in overeating calories during meals in a bid to cover up for the missed meals. Overeating can increase insulin resistance in your body, further leading to weight gain. Research studies revealed that an individual's weight increases when they skip meals due to increased intake of calories per meal and increased abdominal fat (House et al., 2013). Therefore, eat all meals to enhance the normal regulation of your blood sugar levels.

Snack When You're Hungry

Snacking is a vital part of a diet. It decreases hunger in between meals, which keeps you from over-eating your meals. Steer clear from unhealthy snacks as they tend to promote weight gain. Excluding junk food and snacks from your grocery list would be the best way to avoid them.

Properties of healthy snacks include high water and fiber content, while they should be low in fat, calories, and sugars. Fruits, vegetables, nuts, and grains are the best food options to choose from. Some examples of healthy snacks include apples, carrots, nuts, bananas, and raisins. Paring any of the foods with plant-based cheese, puddings, smoothies, yogurts, and hummus helps to reduce your hunger. Snack portions should be limited so that you don't overeat and promote weight gain. Keep them in a small and accessible bag or container that is easy to carry around.

Cook at Home

Invest your time in learning new recipes and healthy cooking techniques. Practice healthy cooking methods, such as steaming, grilling, baking, boiling, air frying, and braising. Remember to steer clear from deep frying. Add healthy, flavorful spices and herbs to garnish and make your food tasty. Continue to explore new and exotic plant-based food. Cooking at home makes you control every ingredient that you consume. Packing your homemade lunch also prevents you from buying unhealthy junk food.

Create a Healthy Food Environment

Your old cravings will inevitably try to crawl into your new plant-based lifestyle. Prepare to respond and overcome them to avoid stressing or giving up. Preparing involves creating an environment that complements a plant-based diet.

Clear out your pantry of animal-based products and unhealthy refined food. If you live with non-plant-based dieters and unhealthy food is in the house, the best way would be to reorganize the food in the pantry and fridge. Place the unhealthy food in top drawers and out of sight, while the healthy food is easily accessible. You could also try to find plant-based restaurants in your area.

Incorporate Supporting Healthy Habits

A healthy lifestyle is not composed of a diet only, but it also includes other complementary habits. Incorporate healthy habits such as exercising and sporting activities to complement your new diet. You will also speed up your weight-loss goals by combining exercise and diet. Meditation or yoga will also help you relax, clear your mind of stress, and be more attentive to the food you decide to eat.

Team Up

Teaming up with a friend, family member, or coworker on the adventure will keep you motivated. You can also consider joining a plant-based diet empowered group in your community or on social media platforms. It will acquire more information and encouragement on how to overcome mishaps, which makes the transition less daunting. A team will provide you with social and emotional support. You can accomplish your goals and celebrate together, which also makes the journey more enjoyable.

Ask for Support

Lifestyle changes can be socially and emotionally overwhelming, so consider consulting with a psychologist. A professional psychologist can help you respond to your emotional challenges. You can also consult a dietitian to help you plan and set attainable goals. A fellow plant-based dieter can also share their struggle and how they overcome the challenges to strengthen your resilience and commitment.

Reward Yourself

Embrace and celebrate all the mini and massive victories, like weekly and monthly goals. Motivate yourself with external rewards such as a new dress, pedicure, or hairstyle that you have always wanted.

Don't Give up

While some experience weight loss in a short period, others take time to see results. If you do not see the results, you expect yet, remain committed because it helps you lose weight sooner or later. You may experience occasional mishaps, but don't give up. It's like dropping a piece of food on the floor, and then you decide to drop the whole plate. Instead, be resilient and aim for consistency, not perfection.

5

THE RECIPES—BREAKFAST

B reakfast is the first and most important meal, which provides the body with energy to start the day. Eating a healthy breakfast with fiber keeps the stomach satiated to prevent overeating, which helps you lose weight and maintain the body you desire. Skipping breakfast increases your blood sugar levels, storage of fat, and the rate of gaining weight (Schlesinger et al., 2018). This is because when you skip your breakfast, the low energy levels in your body will cause you to overeat when you get food. You might even end up eating unhealthy snacks that are high in calories.

Research revealed that eating breakfast also boosts your immune system by increasing gamma-interferon (Beckman and Design, 2003). Gamma-interferon is a protein that has antiviral properties, which induce immune cells to fight diseases. Skipping breakfast was shown to reduce these proteins.

This chapter will highlight the properties that a healthy and nutritious breakfast meal should include. A healthy breakfast limits fat, cholesterol, and sodium intake, while it contains whole grain, fresh fruit, vegetables, and legumes. This chapter also presents various recipes, which will help you when preparing for a plant-based breakfast.

Banana-Blueberry Oats

Banana-blueberry overnight oats are perfect for achieving your weight-loss goals because oats are jam-packed with fiber, iron, and protein, which will make you feel satiated for longer. Banana, blueberries, and coconut milk don't only sweeten the oatmeal; they also add more essential nutrients and minerals. Blueberries, bananas, and oats contain high amounts of antioxidants and vitamin C, which help to boost the immune system. The antioxidants also scavenge free radicals that are oxidative in the body.

The oats can also be stored in the fridge for up to 4 days. Thus, you can save time and pre-make breakfast once and still enjoy it for the next four days. Adding chia seeds provides more protein, fiber, omega-3 fatty acids and improves the texture of the meal to a creamy consistency. The preparation time for this meal is 10 minutes. After leaving the meal overnight in the fridge for at least six hours, you will have one bowl of banana blueberry oats.

What You Need

- Unsweetened coconut, almond, or cashew milk (½ cup)
- Old-fashioned or rolled oats (½ cup)
- Fresh blueberries (½ cup)
- Chia seeds (½ tablespoon)
- Ripe, mashed banana (½)
- Sugar (1 teaspoon)
- Salt (1 pinch)
- Unsweetened flaked coconut (1 tablespoon)

Instructions

1. Combine rolled oats, almond milk, chia seeds, banana, and salt in a container or jar. Add blueberries, seal the lid, and refrigerate overnight for at least six hours.
2. Stir and add a little more milk as the oats may be thicker in the morning. Serve and garnish with chopped nuts to add crunchy texture and flavor. You can store the oats for up to three to four days and use them for other breakfast meals.

Quinoa Cinnamon Bowl

Quinoa is also a low glycemic food, which reduces blood sugar levels and the risk of diabetes. It is also heavy in protein and fiber, which aid weight loss and belly fat. Cinnamon is a calcium, iron, and antioxidant powerhouse, which boosts the immune system and reduces blood pressure, digestive disorders, and blood sugar levels. The recipe also allows topping with more plant-based ingredients, such as nuts, seeds, herbs, and fruits, to provide and balance nutrients in the meal. Interchange your oatmeal by preparing this whole-grain delicious quinoa breakfast bowl using this recipe.

The preparation time for this meal is five minutes. After cooking for 20 minutes using the recipe that is described in this section, you will have two bowls of the cinnamon quinoa bowl.

What You Need

- Uncooked quinoa (½ cup)
- Cinnamon sticks (2)
- Almond milk (1 cup)
- Pure vanilla extract (½ teaspoon)
- Salt (1 pinch)

- Toasted, sliced almonds (¼ cup)
- Toasted, coconut flakes (¼ cup)
- Peaches (¼ cup)
- Raspberries (¼ cup)

Instructions

1. Rinse the quinoa and place them in a saucepan. Add almond milk, two cinnamon sticks, vanilla, and a pinch of salt to the quinoa.
2. Cover the pan and simmer the ingredients at high heat for five minutes. Occasionally stir the quinoa. Reduce the heat and cook for an additional 10 minutes.
3. Remove the saucepan from the heat. Set aside the quinoa for five minutes to allow the grains to absorb the almond milk.
4. Serve the quinoa and top with toasted coconut, almonds, and fruit. If you enjoy it as porridge, add more warm almond milk. The leftover quinoa can be stored for four to five days in the fridge.

Sweet Potato Toast

Sweet potatoes are low in fat but have large amounts of complex carbohydrates and fiber, which restrain you from overeating by keeping you satiated. Smearing your toasted sweet potato with smashed avocado, nut butter, and oil-free hummus will add more flavor and nutrients, like omega-3 fatty acids, calcium, iron, and protein. Dusting cinnamon or garlic powder on top also adds more fiber, calcium, potassium, iron, and vitamins to help balance the meal.

It is also easy and cheap to make as it requires a few ingredients. To change from ordinary toasted bread, follow this recipe and enjoy the tasty and nutritious switch of toasted sweet potato. The formula described here will require you to set aside about 18 minutes for preparation and cooking for you to get four servings.

What You Need

- Large sweet potato (1)
- Mashed avocado (1)
- Almond butter (½ cup)
- Oil-free hummus (1 cup)
- Natural peanut butter (1 cup)
- Banana (4)
- Cinnamon or garlic powder (1 tablespoon)

Instructions

1. Rinse and slice the sweet potato into long ¼ inch slivers.
2. Toast the slices for six to eight minutes until they are gold and crunchy outside while they remain soft inside. You can use a toaster or toaster oven for this.
3. Spread the smashed avocado, nut butter, and oil-free hummus on the toasted sweet potatoes to add flavor. Top with slices of banana and dust with cinnamon or garlic powder to add even more irresistible flavors.

Hummus

While the toasted potato recipe uses hummus as a slather on sweet potatoes, it can also be used as a dip, salad dressing, or savory dish. Hummus is loaded with fiber and proteins, which promote weight loss. It is also versatile as it can be flavored with many ingredients to make it sweet or savory. Consider learning how to prepare hummus at home for its many uses. Also, learn how to use chickpeas that are leftover in just five minutes. The recipe described here will yield one cup of hummus.

What You Need

- Cooked chickpeas (15 ounces)
- Fresh lemon juice (¼)
- Tahini (3 tablespoons)
- Small garlic clove (1)
- Water or aquafaba (3 tablespoons)
- Virgin olive oil (3 tablespoons)
- Salt (½ teaspoon)
- Ground paprika (¼ teaspoon)

Instructions

1. Mix tahini and lemon juice in a food processor for one minute. Stir the mixture while scraping the sides and bottom. Process again for 30 seconds to make the tahini creamier.
2. Mince the garlic and add it along with olive oil and salt to the tahini mixture. Process the mixture for another 30 seconds.
3. Take the cooked chickpeas and rinse them. Add the chickpeas to the mixture in the food processor and process for approximately 2 minutes. Slowly add two to three tablespoons of aquafaba while the mixture is processing until it's smooth and consistent.
4. Serve the hummus with a dash of salt and paprika. You can store the hummus in the fridge in a sealed container for up to one week.

Plant-Based Chickpea Pancake

The chickpea flour is loaded with seven grams of proteins and three grams of fiber per quarter cup. Fiber helps to control hunger and reduce overeating, which promotes the maintenance of belly fat. Toppings and mix-in ingredients of the pancake vary depending on taste. Incorporating plant-based ingredients into the pancake mix and topping adds more flavor and nutrients. This recipe tops cashew cream, hummus, avocado and mix in onion, garlic, black pepper, cinnamon, and kale. Simply set aside 20 minutes for this delicious recipe.

What You Need

- Chickpea flour also called garbanzo flour (½ cup)
- Finely chopped green onion (¼ cup)
- Freshly ground black pepper (⅛ teaspoon)
- Water (¾ cup)
- Garlic powder (¼ teaspoon)
- Fine-grain sea salt (¼ teaspoon)
- Baking powder (¼ teaspoon)
- Finely chopped red pepper (¼ cup)

Instructions

1. Turn on the stove to medium heat and preheat the skillet.
2. Mix the chickpea flour, garlic powder, salt, black pepper, and baking powder in a bowl.
3. Pour in water and whisk for about 15 seconds until the mixture is consistent and airy without clumps. Chop the onions and red pepper into thin and small pieces that cook faster and add them to the mixture.
4. When the pan is hot, lightly spray with plant-based oil.

When you are limiting the intake of oil, use low-fat yogurt, applesauce, or mashed banana to prevent the pancake from sticking.

5. Pour the mixture in batches into the pan depending on the preferred size. Spread the mixture immediately after pouring to cover the floor of the pan. Cook each side for approximately six minutes until it's lightly golden brown and firm to flip. Chickpea pancakes are denser than regular pancakes; therefore, ensure that they are cooked.

6. Serve and garnish the pancakes with avocado, Cinnamon, cashew cream cheese, or your desired plant-based ingredients.

Cashew Cream Cheese

While the previous recipe used cashew cream cheese as a base for topping, it is also used in sweet and savory meals during any time of the day. The nut cheese can be used as a dressing, dip, or spread. Despite being yummy, plant-based cashew cream cheese contains protein, calcium, vitamin B, and fiber.

The fiber reduces cravings, which helps to manage a healthy weight. It also has sufficient healthy omega-3 fatty acids, maintaining cholesterol levels in the blood. There are tons of pre-made plant-based cheese products in stores; however, most of them are packed with unhealthy ingredients and preservatives. Therefore, consider following this three-minute recipe to prepare your own cream cheese at home with no hustle of reading the ingredient list on store-bought packages. The following ingredients yield two cups of cashew cream cheese.

What You Need

- Raw unsalted cashews (2 cups)

- Water (1¼ cups)
- Lemon juice (1 tablespoon)
- Salt (¼ teaspoon)
- Nutritional yeast (3 tablespoons)

Instructions

1. You can choose to soak the cashews in water for about two hours or not. If you do, drain and rinse the nuts thoroughly. When the nuts are soaked, they blend faster and become creamier because of the enhanced softness.
2. Transfer the nuts into the blender bowl with lemon, salt, nutritional yeast, and water. Puree the mixture until it's thick and smooth. Add more water to achieve a creamier consistency. The cream can be stored in the fridge for three to four days.

Cheesy Seitan and Mushroom Sandwich

The breakfast sandwich features seitan, pumpkin seeds, cheese, avocado, and kale, loaded on a toasted English muffin. The English muffin in this recipe is a whole wheat-based product containing high fiber, calcium, phosphorus, magnesium, and selenium contents that promote weight loss. Kale is relatively low in calories but with more fiber, reducing appetite and contributing to weight loss. The preparation time for the sandwich is five minutes. After cooking for 10 minutes using the recipe that is described in this section, you will have two sandwiches.

What You Need

- Seitan ragout (1 cup)

- English muffins (2)
- Baby kale (1 cup)
- Cashew cream cheese (6 tablespoons)
- Vegan mustard (1 tablespoon)
- Mushrooms (1 cup)
- Salt (¼ teaspoon)
- Garlic pepper (¼ teaspoon)

Instructions

1. Place foil on the baking sheet and heat the oven to 400°C while warming the seitan ragout in a pot on the stove.
2. Slice the muffins horizontally and smear mustard on the insides of the bottom halves and cream cheese on the insides of the top halves. Load seitan onto the bottom halves and place all halves on the foil-lined baking sheet. Put the muffins in the oven for about five minutes until they are slightly golden.
3. Remove the muffins from the oven. Rinse and chop the baby kales and mushrooms. Sauté the baby kales and mushrooms in a pan for five minutes and season them with garlic, pepper, and salt to taste. Assemble the halves and add the kales in between the halves and enjoy them when warm.

Plant-Based Tofu Scramble

A vegan tofu scramble is the best to switch from the regular breakfast toast, sandwich, or oatmeal. Tofu is the best ingredient for weight loss because it is low in carbohydrates and cholesterol. Tofu also boosts your daily requirement of protein, calcium, and manganese.

Tofu scramble features a variety of nutritious vegetables and legumes with fiber, satisfying your hunger and promoting a healthy loss of weight. Legumes, like chickpeas or black beans, with vegetables, like broccoli, bell peppers, or tomatoes, taste great with scrambled tofu. You can consider adding mushrooms, seeds, spices, and toasted nuts to add flavor and more nutrients, like omega-3 fatty acids, iron, and vitamins.

You can also top with more plant-based ingredients to balance your nutrients. The meal is also free from gluten and oil to promote a healthy weight. Follow this ten-minute recipe to prepare a tofu scramble that serves two plates using medium-firm or firm tofu. Medium-firm or firm tofu can be crumbled and scrambled without being soggy.

What You Need

- Medium-firm or firm tofu (175 grams)
- Chopped red and green pepper (1/2 cup)
- Chopped mushrooms (½ cup)
- Almond or oat milk (2 tablespoons)
- Chopped broccoli (¼ cup)
- Garlic powder (¼ teaspoon)
- Turmeric (¼ teaspoon)
- Chili powder (½ teaspoon)
- Nutritional yeast (1 tablespoon)
- Ground black pepper (⅛ teaspoon)
- Salt (1 pinch)
- Avocado (1/2)
- Chopped scallions (1 tablespoon)

Instructions

1. Chop your mushroom, broccoli, scallions, green and red peppers into small pieces that will cook faster.

2. Add the vegetables to a pan and cook them on medium heat for approximately seven minutes. Drizzle some water instead of oil to sauté and prevent the vegetables from sticking.

3. Break your tofu into small pieces in a bowl using a masher, fork, or your hands; while cooking the vegetables. Season and mix the tofu in the bowl with spices and plant-based milk.

4. Pour the tofu mixture into the pan with the vegetables and mix by stirring. Add more water or plant-based milk to prevent sticking in the pan. Simmer the scrambled tofu for approximately five minutes and remove it from the heat.

5. Slice an avocado to garnish the tofu scramble.

Oil-Free Chickpea Scramble

Chickpea scramble is another tasty and savory dish loaded with proteins. The meal is low in calories and high in fiber, which helps in weight loss and improves digestion. It also features vegetables for more nutrients, which can be served on the side, like potatoes, tomatoes, and red peppers.

Adding herbal spices to chickpeas, such as garlic, cinnamon, or turmeric, adds antioxidants that help combat diseases. The dish is oil-free, which makes it perfect as a weight loss meal. It also promotes heart health. Chickpea scramble is a versatile dish that tastes well with other ingredients. Thus, adding omega-3 fat sources, such as avocado, would be healthier and tastier. Follow this ten-minute recipe for a guaranteed delicious switch to the tofu scramble, which serves four plates.

What You Need

- Canned or cooked chickpeas (400 grams)

- Lemon juice (2 tablespoons)
- Nutritional yeast (2 tablespoons)
- Garlic powder (1 teaspoon)
- Red bell pepper (½)
- Turmeric powder (½ teaspoon)
- Ground black pepper (¼ teaspoon)
- Salt (¼ teaspoon)
- Hummus (6 tablespoons)
- Mushrooms (½ cup)
- Avocado (1)
- Cherry tomatoes (2)

Instructions

1. Place the chickpeas and lemon juice into a bowl and mash using a fork. Add the hummus, garlic powder, nutritional yeast, salt, and black pepper to the chickpeas and mash again.
2. Transfer the chickpea mixture to a frying pan and cook over medium to high heat until the chickpeas turn golden brown for about five minutes. Stir occasionally to ensure the chickpeas don't stick onto the pan.
3. Rinse, slice, and sauté the mushrooms, peppers, and tomatoes in a separate pan at medium heat for five minutes without oil or any liquid. Remove from heat when the mushrooms turn golden brown.
4. Serve the chickpea scramble with avocado, crispy mushrooms, red pepper, and tomatoes. The chickpea scramble can be sealed in a container and stored in the fridge for up to five days.

Smoothie Bowl

The smoothie bowl is loaded with flavor and nutrients. The smoothie contains tasty clementine and mangoes jam-packed with vitamin C, boosting your immune system to prevent diseases. Incorporating ginger and cinnamon sticks into the smoothie adds taste and antioxidants that help with digestion and boost the immune system. Blending with avocado adds fiber, improves your gut health, and gives the smoothie a thick creamy consistency. Add some seeds or toasted nuts to provide the smoothies with some crunchy texture and nutty flavor. The recipe is versatile, as you can change the ingredients to your liking. Reserve ten minutes of your time to prepare two and a half cups of the smoothie.

What You Need

- Water (¾ cup)
- Frozen Diced mango (1 cup)
- Avocado (⅓ cup)
- Peeled ginger (½ inch)
- Fresh baby spinach (1 cup)
- Peeled clementine (1)
- Almond or peanut butter (3 tablespoons)
- Raspberries, blueberries, or strawberries (1 cup)
- Hemp seeds (1 cup)
- Cinnamon sticks (2)
- Nuts (¼ cup)
- Banana (1)
- Coconut flakes (¼ cup)

Instructions

1. Chop your mangoes, clementine, ginger, baby spinach, and avocado in a bowl.
2. Put the chopped ingredients into a blender and add water, hemp seeds, cinnamon sticks, and vanilla granola. Blend the ingredients at high speed until smooth.
3. Transfer the smoothie into a bowl and garnish with toasted nuts, diced mango, banana slices, or coconut flakes.

Quinoa Breakfast Cookies

Starting the morning with healthy quinoa cookies is energizing and delicious. The cookies are gluten-free and satiating, which keeps you from overeating. They are made with oats, carrots, and quinoa. Carrots, quinoa, and oats are whole grains loaded with protein and fiber, perfect for watching your weight. They are also low in carbohydrates which helps to keep you from gaining weight. The addition of superfoods, such as walnuts, flaxseeds, and pumpkin seeds, make the cookies tastier and healthier by adding more flavor and nutrients, such as omega-3 fatty acids. The recipe requires 15 minutes each for preparation and baking to serve 12 cookies.

What You Need

- Gluten-free oat flour or rolled oats (1 cup)
- Almond milk (1 cup)
- Cooked quinoa (½ cup)
- Baking soda (½ teaspoon)
- Coconut oil (¼ cup)
- Cinnamon (½ teaspoon)
- Sea salt (½ teaspoon)
- Ground flaxseeds (2 tablespoons)

- Finely shredded carrots (1 cup)
- Warm water (5 tablespoons)
- Maple syrup (½ cup)
- Walnuts (¼ cup)
- Pumpkin seeds (¼ cup)
- Dried cranberries (½ cup)

Instructions

1. Take a parchment paper to line the baking sheet and turn on the oven to 190°F for 10 to 15 minutes before baking.
2. Grind the oats using a blender into fine flour. Take one cup of the oat flour and mix in the dry ingredients first: cinnamon, baking powder, shredded carrots, baking soda, and salt into a large bowl.
3. Soak the flax seeds in warm water in a separate bowl and allow them to absorb water and thicken for five minutes.
4. Mix the cooked quinoa, coconut, almond butter, maple syrup, and milk in a separate bowl. Combine the flour mixture, quinoa mixture, and flaxseeds. Add walnuts, cranberries, and pumpkin seeds.
5. Fill a large spoon with the mixture that is prepared for each cookie and place it onto the baking sheet separately. Bake in the oven for 15 to 18 minutes until slightly brown. Remove from the oven and set aside on a wire rack for five minutes, and allow them to cool. These cookies can be kept in a sealed container or frozen.

Healthy Plant-Based Spreads

Spreads are an important part of your breakfast for toast or for adding sweetness to your savory scramble dishes. However, the store-bought products are packed with unhealthy additives, palm oil, refined sugar, gluten, and sodium. To ensure that your spreads are perfectly healthy, follow this recipe to prepare your various plant-based spreads. Like hummus and cashew cheese cream, the spreads are gluten-free and can be topped with vegetables, fruits, nuts, and seeds to make them even healthier. This section provides the recipe to make two different healthy spreads. The spreads are easy and affordable, with a few ingredients. The process is also quick, taking just 5 minutes to prepare a jar of each spread.

Turmeric-Bean Spread

Turmeric in the spread contains a wide range of anti-inflammatory and antioxidant substances, such as curcumin, which boost the immune system. Turmeric also regulates blood sugar levels to prevent the storage of excess fat in the body, thus helping lose and maintain weight. White beans are full of protein and fiber, which also promote a healthy weight.

What You Need

- Canned white beans (1 cup)
- Turmeric powder (1 tablespoon)
- Lemon juice (3 tablespoons)
- Tahini (2 tablespoons)
- Mild or spicy mustard (1 teaspoon)
- Salt (¼ teaspoon)
- Pepper (1/8 teaspoon)
- Onion (½ teaspoon)
- Garlic powder (½ teaspoon)

- Water (5 tablespoons)

Instructions

1. Rinse and drain the beans.
2. Place the entire ingredients in a high-speed blender and process until it's creamy.
3. Add spices and water to make the paste thin and ready for use.

Tahini-Avocado Lemon Spread

Tahini is highly nutritious with antioxidants, which strengthen the immune system. Avocados are high in fiber, which reduces appetite to promote weight loss. A pinch of black pepper in the spread also adds a dash of antioxidants, vitamins, and minerals to start the day.

What You Need

- Ripe avocados (½)
- Tahini (1 teaspoon)
- Lemon juice (½ teaspoon)
- Black pepper (½)

Instructions

1. Mash the avocado with a masher or fork into a creamy paste.
2. Add tahini, lemon juice, spices, and mix to form a paste that is ready to use.

6

THE RECIPES—LUNCH

This chapter will focus on a variety of plant-based recipes that you can have for lunch. The necessary ingredients and quantities will be given for your convenience. Preparation and cooking instructions are provided. By simply looking at the ingredients, you can easily update your shopping list. You could also meal prep for the week and have your meals ready for cooking whenever you desire.

As we discussed earlier, you can obtain numerous benefits from consuming plant-based foods. Some of the benefits include low risks of cardiovascular disease, cancers, and type 2 diabetes. In addition to that, your digestion and skin health will improve. Most of all, plant-based diets have been seen to control weight issues, thereby preventing or reversing the effects of obesity. It is important to note that in order to claim these benefits, you have to be consistent with having plant-based foods. Ensure to always have your lunch so that you keep healthy.

Lunch is vital for providing nourishment and energy to maintain brain and body function throughout the afternoon (provitamil.com, 2010). Furthermore, having lunch reduces stress and offers the necessary break from the day's activities, reducing food cravings. It can be seen that it is crucial to have lunch. It is even more beneficial to have a healthy, plant-based one. Therefore, ensure always to have your plant-based lunches every day. This chapter provides you with many options that could help you in this great endeavor.

The Recipes

There are various recipes that you could try out for lunch. These include the buddha bowl, adzuki bean bowl, stuffed poblano peppers, radish salad, broccoli soup, sesame soba noodles, and vegetarian chili. We will learn about each of these in this section.

Buddha Bowl

According to Katherine Sacks, in her 2017 *Epicurious* article, the name of this lunch dish stems from the way Buddha used a large bowl to collect whatever alms that villagers could share in the various villages he was staying in (loveandlemons.com, 2017). The Buddha bowl will take you approximately 15 minutes to prepare the ingredients and 20 minutes of cooking time. In 35 minutes, you will have your lunch ready to serve four people. Let's take a look at the ingredients and cooking instructions in greater detail.

What You Need

- Cubed sweet potato (1, preferably a large one)
- Red radishes (2) or watermelon radish (1)
- Shredded red cabbage (1 cup)

- Medium-sized carrots (2)
- Freshly cracked black pepper and sea salt
- Lemon juice (a squeeze will do)
- Hemp or sesame seeds (2 tablespoons)
- Chopped kale leaves (8)
- Cooked quinoa or brown rice (2 cups)
- Cooked lentils or chickpeas (1 cup)
- Any fermented veggie or sauerkraut (3/4 cup)
- Extra-virgin oil
- Microgreens (optional)
- For serving, you can add Turmeric Tahini Sauce

Instructions

1. Heat the oven to 400°F prior to lining a large baking sheet with parchment paper.
2. Drizzle the sweet potatoes with olive oil, pepper, and salt. Spread the sweet potatoes onto the baking sheet and roast for 20 minutes, or until the potatoes have become golden brown.
3. Preferably on a mandoline, slice the radish into thin rounds and peel the carrots into ribbons, using a vegetable peeler.
4. Toss the carrots, shredded cabbage, and radish slices with a squeeze of lemon. Put this aside.
5. In a large bowl, put the kale leaves and toss with little pinches of salt and a squeeze of lemon. Massage the kale leaves with your hands until they are soft and flaccid such that they appear to have reduced by half.
6. Arrange single bowls with the chickpeas, brown rice, radishes, carrots, kale, sweet potatoes, cabbages, sesame seeds, sauerkraut, and microgreens, if using any. Add pepper and salt for seasoning. You can serve the Buddha bowl with the Turmeric Tahini Sauce.

Tips to Spice-Up Your Buddha Bowl

You can have your buddha bowl as given in the recipe mentioned above. Please note that it is also possible to make some changes to the dish and still get the health benefits of the plant-based lunch that you desire. And you also get a different taste of the same dish. Let's delve deeper into the options.

- **Change up the veggies:** Instead of the sweet potato, you could try regular potatoes or roasted butternut squash. You might as well try a different kind of roasted veggie such as roasted broccoli, asparagus, cauliflower, beets, or Brussels sprouts. Another option that can present you with an altogether different taste would be to cook the veggies in another way. Instead of leaving the kale raw, you could sauté or steam it, simmer the sweet potatoes, or roast the carrots.
- **Vary the grain:** Quinoa, couscous, or farro can replace the rice. You can add these substitutes for a different and healthy option.
- **Try another pickle:** Sauerkraut can be replaced by jalapeños or pickled red onion. Try these if sauerkraut is not readily available to you.
- **Add in a different protein:** For your protein shift, you could try lentils, edamame, or black beans. Any other type of beans would be great as well. You could add tempeh, crispy tofu, or roasted chickpeas to top your grain bowl.
- **Change up the sauce:** Apart from the Tahini sauce, any other different sauce will do. Options can range from lemon vinaigrette, peanut sauce, cilantro lime dressing, drizzles of sesame oil and tamari, or hummus.

Stuffed Poblano Peppers

The preparation time for stuffed poblano peppers is 20 minutes. Cook time will be about 20 minutes. Therefore, in approximately 40 minutes, your stuffed poblano peppers will be ready to serve four people. We will look at the necessary ingredients and cooking instructions in this section.

What You Need

- Small pieces of cauliflower florets (1 heaped cup)
- Chopped scallions or diced red onion (⅓ cup)
- Medium-sized poblano peppers (4)
- For drizzling, you will need extra-virgin olive oil
- Diced, red bell pepper (½ cup)
- Crushed garlic clove (1)
- Cooked, drained, and rinsed black beans (1 cup)
- Cooked brown rice (1 cup)
- Coriander (½ cup)
- Cumin (½ teaspoon)
- Oregano (½ teaspoon)
- Fresh spinach (3 cups)
- Lime juice (2 tablespoons). Wedges can be added when serving
- Tomatillo salsa (1/4 cup)
- Ground black pepper
- Sea salt

Instructions

1. After preheating the oven to 400°F, use parchment paper to line a baking sheet.
2. Cut the peppers into two equal parts and take out the ribbing and seeds. Put them on the baking sheet and

drizzle with olive oil. Sprinkle with pinches of pepper and salt before roasting for 15 minutes, with the cut side up.

3. Heat a tablespoon of olive oil in a big frying pan over medium heat. Add the cauliflower, onion, cumin, red pepper, oregano, coriander, half a teaspoon of salt, black pepper, and garlic. Cook for about five to eight minutes until the cauliflower is slightly brown and the onion is soft.

4. Remove the frying pan from the heat and stir in the rice, black beans, lime juice, tomatillo salsa, and spinach. Taste and alter the seasonings according to your preference.

5. Put the filling into the peppers prior to baking for 15 minutes.

6. Serve with cilantro, green chili cashew cream, tomatillo salsa, lime, and avocado slices on the side.

Different Versions of the Stuffed Poblano Peppers

Depending on your preferences, there are different ways in which you can have your stuffed poblano peppers, apart from the recipe mentioned above. It could be totally plant-based, or you could add some cheese. Let's explore the options in depth.

- **Entirely plant-based:** You could top the peppers with guacamole or avocado slices, chili lime cashew cream, and additional tomatillo salsa. Cilantro lime dressing, chipotle sauce, or cashew sour cream would also be great options.

- **Melty cheese on top:** If you like, you could top your stuffed peppers with a layer of shredded cheese prior to baking them. Let them bake until the cheese melts and becomes brownish.

- **Add some cheese to the filling:** A mixture of crumbled cottage and feta cheeses can be stuffed into the peppers before adding the stuffing. Bake them and add your favorite sauce.

Radish Salad

The radish salad is remarkable when the radishes are crispy and a little sweet. The preparation time is about 15 minutes, while the cooking time is approximately 10 minutes. In about 25 minutes, your radish salad will be ready. Four servings can be obtained from this recipe.

What You Need

- Fresh mint leaves (1/4 cup)
- Pine nuts (1/4 cup)
- Radish green pesto, or any other (1/4 cup)
- Thinly sliced red radishes (2-3)
- Shaved pecorino or Parmesan (2 tablespoons) (optional)
- Freshly ground black pepper and sea salt
- Lemon juice (optional)
- Capers (1 tablespoon)
- Lemon vinaigrette (1/4 cup)
- Quartered or halved, roasted radishes (9)
- Cooked, drained, and rinsed navy bean

Instructions

1. Mix two tablespoons of the Lemon Vinaigrette with beans in a medium bowl.
2. Put the salad on a platter and add beans, sliced raw

radishes, pine nuts, roasted radishes, capers, and spoonfuls of pesto.

3. Drizzle with the rest of the dressing and top with pecorino and fresh mint. Sprinkle more pepper and salt to taste, as well as additional squeezes of lemon if preferred.

Some Tips on Radish Salad Recipe

The recipe mentioned above for radish salad is an excellent variation of many others that you could try. Different ingredients can be added, and the timing for adding the mint leaves may as well be altered to produce a new taste altogether. Let's look at the different variations in this section.

- **Maintain the Crunch of Roasted Radishes:** If the radishes are too soft, they won't blend well with the creamy white beans. To maintain the crunch, ensure to roast them for only 10-15 minutes.
- **Make it in Advance:** This is a great recipe when it comes to making it ahead of time because the ingredients are readily available. You could pack it for a picnic or lunch. If possible, add the mint leaves just before having the salad in order to maintain their freshness.
- **Make Some Variations:** The recipe is fantastic, as given above, but you could make some great changes too. Toss in some arugula; a handful will do. You could also use French green lentils instead of white beans. In addition to the mint, some fresh herbs such as tarragon, basil, or thyme could be used. Adding in some crumbled feta cheese could be useful as well. Watermelon radishes, Persian cucumbers, or Easter egg radishes could replace the sliced red radishes. The

other option could be to stir in chopped roasted asparagus.

Broccoli Soup

The rich and creamy broccoli soup takes 15 minutes to prepare the ingredients and 35 minutes of cook time. After 50 minutes, four servings of this nutritious soup will be ready. Let's get more details on the ingredients and how to cook the broccoli soup.

What You Need

- Broccoli diced stems and chopped florets (1 lb)
- Apple cider vinegar (1½ teaspoons)
- Raw cashews (½ cup)
- Dijon mustard (½ teaspoon)
- Crushed garlic cloves (4)
- Cubed bread for croutons (3 cups)
- Vegetable broth (3 cups)
- Small, diced yukon gold potato (1 cup)
- Fresh dill (¼ cup)
- Sea salt (¾ teaspoon)
- Fresh lemon juice (1 tablespoon)
- Freshly pounded black pepper
- Chopped carrots (⅓ cup)
- Diced, yellow onion (1 small)
- Chopped celery (½ cup)

Instructions

1. Heat the oven to 350°F prior to lining two small baking sheets with parchment paper.
2. Heat the oil in a Dutch oven or a large pot over

medium heat. Add the carrots, celery, onion, broccoli stems, pepper, and salt, then sauté for approximately 10 minutes, until softened. Put in the potatoes and garlic, then stir. Afterward, add the broth and simmer for about 20 minutes until the potatoes are soft. Leave to slightly cool.

3. Reserve a cup of the broccoli florets that you will roast as a topping for the soup. Steam the remainder of the florets in a steaming basket over a pot with about an inch of water. Bring the water to a boil, cover the florets and let them steam for five minutes until the broccoli is soft.

4. In the meantime, place the bread cubes and the reserved broccoli florets on the baking sheets. Toss with a pinch of salt and a drizzle of olive oil until the broccoli is tender and the bread is crusty on its edges. This will take around 10 to 15 minutes.

5. Move the soup to the blender and put in the apple cider vinegar, mustard, and cashews. Blend until creamy. Add the steamed broccoli florets, lemon juice, and dill, ensuring that you pulse until the broccoli is mixed in but still lumpy. The soup should ideally be thick, but you can add about half a cup of water to thin it to your preferred thickness.

6. Season to your desired taste and serve the soup in bowls, with the roasted croutons and broccoli on top.

Tips on Broccoli Soup

Apart from the recipe mentioned above on broccoli soup, other changes can be made, and the result would still be exceptional. The soup could be topped with something crunchy, or you could avoid too much blending of the broccoli. Let's get more details on how to obtain different varieties of the same soup.

- **Add something crunchy:** Crunchy garnishes add some textural contrast to food. Roasted broccoli florets and homemade croutons that are added to the already-simmering soup will result in a delicious soup.
- **Avoid blending the broccoli too much:** To have a good soup texture, avoid blending the broccoli too much. You can blend the celery, potatoes, broccoli stalks, onions, and carrots to complete smoothness, but ensure to simply pulse in the steamed florets.
- **Avoid skipping the dill:** Even if you don't like dill, I recommend considering it in this recipe. It mimics the flavor of cheddar cheese.

Sesame Soba Noodles

Originally from Japan, soba noodles are made from buckwheat flour. They have a slick, soft texture and a nutty flavor. Sesame soba noodles require 10 minutes for ingredient preparation and 10 minutes, cook time. In approximately 20 minutes, about two to four servings will be ready for consumption. Let's have more details on the ingredients and the instructions for cooking the sesame soba noodles.

What You Need

First with the dressing

- Toasted sesame oil (½ teaspoon)
- Grated garlic clove (1)
- Grated ginger (1 teaspoon)
- Rice vinegar (¼ cup)
- Tamari (2 tablespoons). You can add more for serving

Then the noodles

- Soba noodles (6 ounces)
- Blanched snap peas (2 cups)
- Sliced avocados (2)
- Fresh mint leaves (¼ cup)
- Edamame (¼ cup)
- Sesame seeds
- Squeezes of lemon
- Very thinly sliced red radishes (2) or watermelon radish (1)
- Sesame oil (for drizzling)

Instructions

1. To make the dressing, mix the vinegar, sesame oil, tamari, garlic, and ginger. Then set aside.
2. Bring an unsalted pot of water to a boil and cook the soba noodles as instructed on the package. Drain and rinse well in the cold, running water so that you remove the starches that might cause clumping. Thoroughly mix the dressing with the noodles before splitting the mixture into about four bowls. Squeeze the lemon juice over the avocado slices and add to the bowls, together with the edamame, snap peas, mint, and radish. Sprinkle with sesame seeds and drizzle with more sesame oil or tamari, if preferred.

Adzuki Bean Bowl

Adzuki beans are a type of delicious, small beans that cook fast because of their size. The preparation time for this bowl is 20 minutes, and the cooking time is 30 minutes. In approximately 50 minutes, your adzuki bean bowl will be ready to serve four people.

What You Need

- Small carrots that have been shaved with a vegetable peeler (3)
- Sliced avocados (2)
- Sesame seeds (2 tablespoons). You can add more when serving
- Sliced sugar snap peas (1 cup)
- Cooked brown rice (1 cup)
- Chopped fresh cilantro leaves (2 tablespoons). More can be added when serving.
- Cook, drain, and rinse adzuki beans (1½ cups).
- Freshly sliced red chili (1 small one)
- Sliced, Napa cabbage head (6½ cups)

Instructions

Start by making the dressing as follows:

1. Whisk together olive oil, rice vinegar, miso, sesame oil, and tamari in a small bowl.
2. Mix the carrots, cabbage, sesame seeds, and snap peas with a quarter of a cup of the dressing in a large bowl.
3. Fold the cilantro in the cabbage salad before serving. Split equal parts of the cabbage salad, rice, avocados, and beans into four bowls. Use more dressing for drizzling and sprinkle with chili, to taste. You could also add some more sesame and cilantro seeds, according to your preference.

Vegetarian Chili

The vegetarian chili is an easy-to-make, hearty, and spicy meal which takes about 45 minutes to be ready. Its preparation time is 10 minutes, while the cooking time is 35 minutes. This recipe serves six to eight people. We will learn more about preparing vegetarian chili in this section, from the ingredients to the cooking instructions.

What You Need

- Chopped yellow onion (1 small one)
- Diced red bell pepper (1)
- Extra-virgin olive oil (2 tablespoons)
- Crushed garlic cloves (2)
- Drained and rinsed pinto beans can (1 weighs 14-ounces)
- Diced fire-roasted tomatoes can (1 weighs 14-ounces)
- Drained and rinsed red beans can (1 weighs 14-ounces)
- Broth or water (1 cup)
- Frozen or fresh corn kernels (1 cup)
- Sea salt (1/2 teaspoon)
- Lime juice (1 tablespoon). You can add wedges for serving
- Freshly pounded black pepper
- Diced chipotle peppers from canned chipotles in adobo (3), plus sauce (3 tablespoons)

Instructions

1. Heat the oil in a huge pot using medium heat. Put in the onion, little pinches of pepper and salt, then stir. Cook for five minutes until the onion is semi-transparent before putting in red pepper and garlic. Stir and cook for five to eight minutes until soft, ensuring that you appropriately reduce the heat as required.
2. Add the beans, tomatoes, chipotles, water, corn, adobo

sauce, salt, a few grinds of pepper, and corn. Cover and leave to simmer on low heat for 25 minutes, ensure to stir occasionally till the chili soup has become thick.

3. Add in the lime juice and season to your desired taste. Serve with your favorite toppings.

7

THE RECIPES—DINNER

W hen you start eating a plant-based diet, you might feel like the change is just too much for you to be able to cope with. Alternatively, you might even think that you will be fine. No matter what you are thinking, the truth is that your success will mainly depend on the mindset that you will create or adopt as you embark on your new journey. Creativity is key in this game. The better you are at varying your plant-based dishes, the lower the chances that you will give up along the way. This is why this chapter focuses on providing you with different dinner recipes that will spice up your eating routines. Before we get on to recipes, let's look at some of the reasons why you should have dinner as part of your meal routines.

Importance of Dinner

Dinner is an important and indispensable meal that you should have each day. That is why it is essential to carefully prepare this meal, giving special attention to the ingredients that you use. It is crucial for you to know why this meal is that important, and we will address this in this section. Dinner is usually the only meal that families enjoy together in many homes, considering the busy schedules that lace the twenty-first century. Both parents and children have busy mornings and afternoons, making it difficult for them to enjoy breakfast and lunch together. Therefore, sharing your dinner with others simply makes it special.

Aiding Good Sleep and Digestion

It is easy to assume that what you eat at dinner is more important than the time you eat it. On the contrary, these two aspects are both important. The time that you eat your dinner affects how much you get out of the meal in terms of nutrition. Ideally, it is recommended that you have your dinner as close to sunset as possible. The later you have it, the heavier it becomes in your body. Unfortunately, many people tend to eat their dinner late, and desisting from that eating pattern is worth the while. Eating your dinner late is associated with inefficient digestion as well as poor quality and quantity of sleep. Late dinners are also linked with volatile dreams (Kannan, 2020). Ideally, you should have your dinner before 7 p.m., and then staying awake for about two hours will make you feel light and healthy, apart from enhancing better sleep.

Causing a Good Ripple Effect for Other Meals

When you are able to enjoy a good sleep after having a good dinner at the right time, you are in a better position to plan well for other meals of the day. This way, you can better stick to your plant-based diet. Poor sleep can lead to compromised concentration. There are even greater chances that you might slide back to the foods that are prohibited in the plant-based diet. Suppose you wake up late and still feel sleepy; you might just grab a ready-made animal product from the fridge and eat. This is more probable when you are staying with other people who do not subscribe to the plant-based diet like you. Simply put, a good dinner served at the right time causes a positive ripple effect that will see you enjoy great meals with esteem throughout the day.

Controlling Metabolism

A proper dinner helps to improve the rate and efficiency of your metabolism. When metabolic functions are more efficient, weight loss endeavors are easier to realize. A well-prepared dinner with the right ingredients helps balance the sugar levels in the blood and the endocrine system.

Providing Your Body With Energy

Your body will always need energy, even when you are sleeping. If you skip your dinner, your body won't be able to have enough energy to sustain all the energy-consuming processes that take place while you are sleeping. Nearly all the processes that occur within the body require specific amounts of energy. Dinner is the source of all the vitamins, minerals, and other nutrients that will keep you going until your next breakfast. Eating a healthy dinner does not result in weight gain. This notion is based on the fact that humans tend to burn more calories while they are asleep than when they are sitting and watching some cartoons.

More Tips for Planning Your Dinner

Check your mood and health before you prepare your dinner. A well-prepared dinner might be all you need to address some discrepancies in your health. Let's explore some cases that you can address by incorporating the right ingredients in your dinner.

Are You Experiencing Inflammation-Related Pain?

Inflammatory conditions that are coupled with pain can make your night unenjoyable. A relevant dinner can be all you need to become more relaxed as the night passes. Add in some plant-based foods that have remarkable anti-inflammatory attributes. Think of green lentils, yellow pumpkin, ginger, coriander, ginger, and even black pepper. Ginger is helpful in suppressing triggers for swelling and pain.

Are You Struggling With Poor Sleep and Volatile Dreams?

If you are having problems with your sleep, you can correct this by having the appropriate dinner. Volatile dreams and unstable sleep can be associated with compromised liver health and poor digestion. Therefore, the dinner that you need in such a case should be liver rejuvenating. Traditional medicine suggests that bitter greens can enhance the health of the liver. Therefore, green leafy vegetables are a great addition to our dinner in this case. These vegetables contain magnesium that improves better sleep.

When you are going through a stressful period, your body tends to digest food much more quickly than when everything is normal. The same applies when there is a sugar imbalance in your body. To stabilize the digestion process and reduce the food transit time, wholesome meals that include carrots and broccoli will certainly do you good.

Are You Fighting With Psychological Stress and Anxiety?

Mental disturbances linked to stress, depression, and anxiety require that you become more careful about what you eat, including your dinner. Ideally, you should prioritize foods that have positive effects on your brain and overall health. Such foods support the nervous system. Some of such foods improve the secretion of hormones like serotonin and dopamine. Serotonin is also referred to as the 'happiness' hormone, while dopamine is called the 'feel-good hormone. These tag names are quite self-explanatory. Dopamine regulates your mind, movement, and mood, thereby making you feel good. On the other hand, serotonin oversees your digestion, mood, and sleep.

If you are going through anxiety or stress, Shiitake mushrooms are a great addition to your dinner because they contain phytochemicals that enhance your resilience to stress. Also, consider tofu, snow peas, and sesame seeds. Tofu contains good amounts of tryptophan, which improves better sleep quality. However, before you take tofu, make sure you don't have hormonal issues. Otherwise, you would have to replace the tofu with other plant-based foods that are rich in proteins.

Recipes

Now that you have a better understanding of various aspects surrounding your dinner meals let's look at some recipes that you can add to the ones you already have. Variety will remove boredom, thereby making it easier for you to maintain consistency. Not only will you gain the nutritional advantage that the variety of recipes will give you, but you will also give your taste buds the opportunity to enjoy.

Mediterranean Quinoa and Chickpea Salad

This salad is a combination of unique Mediterranean flavors that come from the ingredients that are used in this recipe. This dish is excellent as a side dish. However, you can also use it as the main dish if you add tempeh, tofu, or tortilla. This recipe includes quinoa and chickpeas as some of the main ingredients. These two ingredients are rich sources of protein, so their addition makes the whole dish super nutritious.

What You Need

- Chickpeas (1 can)
- Cooked quinoa (1½ cup)
- Olive oil (1 teaspoon)
- Quartered cherry tomatoes (1 cup)
- Small purple onion (½ bulb)
- Black pepper (⅓ teaspoon)
- Fresh lemon juice (1 tablespoon)
- Salt (1½ teaspoon)
- Green, black, or kalamata olives (10)
- Red wine vinegar (2 teaspoons)
- Balsamic vinegar (1 teaspoon)
- Fresh Basil leaves (1½ cup)

Instructions

1. If your quinoa is dry, you should remove its outer coating, which is bitter. Do this by rinsing them under running water for at least one minute.
2. Put the quinoa in the pan and add three cups of water, together with some salt. Cover the pan and let the contents boil.
3. Cut the onions, tomatoes, basil leaves, olives, and other ingredients in your list that need to be chopped before use.
4. Carefully open a chickpea can and wash them using running water. The liquid from the chickpea can make a great aquafaba, so you can keep it if you wish.
5. Put all the ingredients that you cut in (3) above into a bowl. Also, add the chickpeas and quinoa. Combine everything with vinegar, peppers, olive oil, fresh lemon juice, and more salt.
6. Seve your salad along with tortilla wraps, fresh bread, or any other main dish of your choice.

White Bean Soup

If you want to enjoy a vegetable soup that is coupled with sautéed vegetables, this is the perfect dish for you. This is an easy dish to make and can appetize you with the colorful sight of the white beans and tomatoes dipped in vegetable and tomato broth. The incredible flavors will keep you wanting more of this dish for your special dinners. This dish is a great way to keep yourself unavailable to unhealthy, calorie-rich animal foods that cause you to gain weight. You will need about an hour to prepare this dish.

What You Need

- Olive oil (2 tablespoons)
- Large diced carrots (2)
- Chopped kale (3 cups)
- Vegetable broth (4 cups)
- Dried thyme, oregano, and basil (1 tablespoon each)
- Minced garlic (2 cloves)
- Finely diced, small yellow onion (1)
- Diced celery stalks (2)
- Cannellini beans (1 can 15 oz)
- Fire-roasted diced tomatoes (1 can 15 oz)
- Diced zucchini (2)
- Red pepper flakes (¼ teaspoon)
- Tomato paste (2 tablespoons)
- Black pepper (1/2 teaspoon)
- Salt (1 teaspoon)

Instructions

1. Prepare your vegetables. Dice the tomatoes, onions, zucchini, and carrots. Chop the kale.

2. To prepare the sauté vegetables, add onion, olive oil, carrots, and celery into a large pot or dutch oven. Also, add a little salt and let this cook on medium heat for about five minutes. Add zucchini and garlic into the pot and cook for three more minutes.

3. Now, it's time to add the liquids to the sauté vegetables. Add the cannellini beans, tomato paste, diced tomatoes, vegetable broth, and all your seasonings. Cover the pot and allow the soup to simmer for not more than 30 minutes on low-medium heat. Be sure to stir occasionally.

4. Completely remove the heat before stirring in your chopped kale.

5. Taste the soup before serving it. That's the only way you can determine whether your soap needs more seasoning or flavoring. If your soap requires more salt, just add a pinch and stir it in until the flavor gets to your desired level. Simmer the soup again.

6. Serve and enjoy!

Chickpea and Avocado Salad in Collard Wraps

This is one of the unique plant-based recipes you should try, especially if you are still new to the "green" diet. It is also very simple to prepare. Are you scared of the bitterness in collard? There is no need to worry because the flavor of collard leaves is relatively mild. Moreover, the avocados and chickpeas flavors will blend in and cover up that of the collard leaves. This protein and fiber-rich dish won't take more than 10 minutes of your time to prepare.

What You Need

- Ripe avocado (1)

- Drained and rinsed chickpeas (15-ounce can)
- Diced, large bell pepper (½)
- Diced medium stalk celery (1)
- Pepper (¼ teaspoon)
- Collard leaves
- Diced medium carrot (1)
- Finely chopped cilantro (¼ cup)
- Juiced lemon(1)
- Salt (½ teaspoon)

Instructions

1. Mash the avocado in a small- or medium-sized bowl
2. Get a large bowl and add the chickpeas. Also, mash the chickpeas using a fork or a potato masher. Stir in the bell pepper, celery, and carrot. When these appear well-mixed, add cilantro, lemon juice, mashed avocado, pepper, and salt. Mix well until all the ingredients are combined well. You have just made your salad.
3. Place one collard leaf on a cutting board. Measure about half a cup of the chickpea salad and place it on the center of the flat collard leaf. Fold the edges of the leaf in before rolling the leaf so that it assumes the shape of a burrito.
4. Repeat the procedure to make collard wraps that match the amount of chickpea salad that you made.
5. Put your collard wraps in an air-tight container and store them in the fridge for not more than five days.

Lentil Vegetable Soup

The lentil vegetable soup is one of the most customizable dishes in a plant-based diet. You can easily alter it to meet your needs and taste. The dish is also a great source of plant-based nutrients to help you lose weight and feel healthy.

What You Need

- Medium carrots (2)
- Vegetable broth (4 cups)
- Yellow onion (1)
- Uncooked brown/green lentils (1 cup)
- Dried basil or any other herb that you prefer (1½ teaspoons)
- Garlic (4 cloves)
- Diced or fire-roasted tomatoes (15 oz. can)
- Mushrooms (6 oz.)
- Fresh baby spinach (1 cup)
- Zucchini (1)
- Salt to taste

Instructions

1. Dice the onion.
2. Place your stockpot over medium to high heat and add the diced onion. Sauté Use the no-oil technique for about 8 minutes. You only need three tablespoons of vegetable broth or water for this sauté method. If you notice that the pan is drying out or the onions are sticking to the pan, just add a little more water or vegetable broth.
3. As you sauté the onions, dice the carrots and zucchini, slice the mushrooms, and mince the garlic.
4. Once the onion appears semi-transparent, add the zucchini, garlic, mushrooms, dried basil, and carrots. Mix well and sauté for at least two minutes.

5. Put in the diced tomatoes, along with the vegetable broth.
6. Bring the contents of the pot to a light boil by increasing the heat to high.
7. Rinse the lentils using running water and carefully drain them before adding them to the pot. Stir well.
8. Lower the heat and cover the pot. Leave the pot contents to simmer lightly for about 30 minutes. The lentils should become tender in the process. Be sure to add more vegetable broth or water if the pot dries out.
9. Chop the spinach and add it to the pot in the last five minutes of cooking. Add salt to taste.
10. Serve your dish together with cilantro, basil, or fresh chopped parsley.

Chickpea Curry

This meal is packed with fiber, protein, and iron. Besides, it's exceptionally easy to prepare. Chickpeas also contain manganese, selenium, and folate, whose health benefits are what you need in your weight-loss journey. The nutrients from chickpeas help regulate blood sugar, aid digestion and reduce the risk of heart disease and cancer. Chickpeas also stay in your gut for longer, which makes them helpful in avoiding overeating that leads to weight loss. After just 25 minutes of preparing, your chickpea curry will be ready for you to enjoy.

What You Need

- Basmati rice (½ cup)
- Olive oil (1 tablespoon)
- Curry paste (1 or 2 teaspoons)
- Water (1 cup)
- Low-fat coconut milk (1 can)

- Onions (2)
- Chickpeas (1 can)
- Medium tomatoes (2 or 3)
- Fresh basil (1 cup)
- Lime (½)
- Garlic (3 cloves)
- Soy sauce (1 or 2 tablespoons)
- Salt (2 pinches)

Instructions

1. Add the water, rice, and one pinch of salt into a pot. Heat the water in the pot and begin to boil, after which you should reduce the heat to low and cook further for about ten more minutes. Be sure to close the pot with a lid once the water starts boiling.
2. As the rice boils, cut the basil, garlic, onions, and juice the lime.
3. Add oil into a large pan on low-medium heat. Add the onions and stir them until they become soft and translucent. This should take approximately five minutes. Add the garlic into the pan and cook for a minute more.
4. Add the curry paste together with the milk and stir continuously until the curry dissolves. Add one pinch of salt and taste. If you feel you need a stranger flavor of the curry, you can add one more teaspoon.
5. Get the rinsed and drained chickpeas and add them into the pan. Also, add soy sauce and cook on medium heat for about five minutes until the curry boils. Don't let it burn; otherwise, you should reduce the cooking heat at once.
6. Now, add the basil, tomatoes, soy sauce, lime juice, and gently simmer the curry again for two more minutes.

7. Taste again to determine if you need more soy sauce. If need be, add brown sugar or another tablespoon of soy sauce. Stir again.
8. At this point, the rice should be well-cooked, too. Simply use a fork to loosen it and give it a fluffy feel or appearance.
9. Serve your dinner with rice and curry. You can serve the meal with naan bread as an optional side dish.

Loaded Sweet Potatoes

This is one of the recipes you can prepare during the fall when sweet potatoes are available in abundance. In this recipe, the sweet potatoes are loaded with various greens, veggies, and other plant-based foods in their brilliant colors. This implies that this meal comes with a variety of nutrients and antioxidants that your body certainly needs, especially when you are channeling all your energy toward losing weight. Preparing this dish does not demand much of your precious time and energy.

What You Need

- Medium-sized sweet potatoes (4)
- Wild rice blend (½ cup)
- Shelled and unsalted pumpkin seeds (3 tablespoons)
- Dried cranberries (½ cup)
- Cinnamon (½ teaspoon)
- Balsamic vinegar (½ teaspoon)
- Water (3 tablespoons)
- Whole white mushrooms
- Medium-sized yellow onion (½)
- Sugar (1 tablespoon)
- Tahini (¼ cup)

Instructions

1. Begin by baking the sweet potatoes because they will take a lot of time. To do so, preheat the oven to 425°F. Carefully rinse the sweet potatoes under running water before stabbing holes in them. The purpose of this is to release steam and shorten the cooking time.

2. Place the sweet potatoes on a baking sheet, which you should put in the oven for about 45 minutes. Depending on the oven that you use, you might need more or less time to bake the sweet potatoes. Whatever the case might be, just stab into the sweet potatoes; if they are soft throughout, then they are fully baked.

3. Prepare for the other steps while the sweet potatoes are baking—Cook the wild rice blend according to the instructions given on the packaging. Generally, the water to rice ratio should be 2:1—Cook the rice for 25 minutes.

4. Chop the quarter mushrooms and onions. Place a pan on medium heat, add olive oil, and cook the vegetables until the onions are semi-transparent and mushrooms are soft. This should take approximately about 10 minutes.

5. Add the well-cooked rice blend to the pan containing onions and mushrooms, and immediately turn off the heat. Also, add the dried cranberries and thoroughly mix all the pan contents together.

6. Cover the rice blend with a lid to maintain warm temperatures as you finish baking the sweet potatoes.

7. Start making the tahini dressing. To do this, add tahini, maple syrup, balsamic vinegar, and cinnamon into a bowl. Gradually add a tablespoon of water at a time, continuously stirring until you reach the desired

consistency, which is dependent on personal preferences.

8. Transfer the completely baked sweet potatoes from the oven to a cutting board. Hold the sweet potato in place using a fork while you cut it in a longitudinal direction to open a gap in which you will add your filling.

9. Scoop the filling into the center of the opened gap on the sweet potatoes. Top the filling with the tahini dressing and some pumpkin seeds.

10. Serve your dish, and enjoy!

8

THE RECIPES—SNACKS

C hoosing a healthy snack can be a huge challenge for people who are trying to take care of themselves or are trying to watch their weight. For some reason, snacks have developed a bad image because they are viewed as an unnecessary part of the diet. They, however, can be an essential part of the diet because they can provide you with energy in the middle of the day or during those times when you exercise. Healthy snacks in between meals can also help by decreasing your hunger, such that when you eat, you do not overdo it. The fuller you feel at mealtime, the less you will eat.

There are many healthy snacks to choose from. The only challenge you may have is identifying which snack can be dubbed as healthy and which cannot. Once you read through this book, you will be enlightened on what constitutes healthy eating between meals. It is vital to remember that not all snacks will contribute to your health. You should try by all means possible to decrease the number of unhealthy snacks that you take. For people watching their weight, you will find that most of the weight is gained from the food eaten in-between meals than from the food eaten at meals.

Tips to Help You Limit Junk Food

Sometimes you need a strategy to help you get over unhealthy eating when it comes to snacks. Usually, we tend to eat a lot of the stuff that is available in our houses. Because of that, you need to ensure that almost all the food you have around is healthy. Give yourself a whole lot of healthy options. The best way to avoid unhealthy snacks is not to have them in your house. Here are a few other tips to help you to maintain healthy snacking.

- Whenever possible, pack your snacks in small plastic bags or containers so that they are easy for you to carry around in your bag or backpack. Packaging your snacks before you need to eat them is advisable because it helps you control the portions. You just plan ahead for your day, and always prepare the snacks that you will eat during the course of the day so that you will not fall for any other unhealthy options.

- You must always limit junk food snacks. Ice cream, candy, chips, and cake are notable examples of unhealthy snacks that have to be kept minimal. Avoid having these foods in your house. You may have them once in a while, but you should ensure that they are not lying around at your disposal at any given time because you will end up indulging.

- Remember not to be so uptight. It is alright to have an unhealthy snack here and there. If you are too hard on yourself, you may end up sneaking on these foods, and you will end up over-indulging, which is not a good thing. Remember that balance and moderation is key. Unhealthy snacks eaten in moderation and in balance with healthy food will not be as harmful.

- For every unhealthy snack, try to find out if there is a healthy option. For example, you can replace the candy dish with a fruit bowl. There are almost always some healthy options in regard to our snacks. If a healthier replacement is available, go for it.

- If you have unhealthy snacks like cookies and candy in the house, try storing them far from reach or somewhere where they cannot be seen. This can be something like a high shelf or a lockable cupboard. You can store ice cream, expel it at the back of the freezer, and have healthier foods upfront. Not having unhealthy snacks in your sight is very helpful.

- Suppose you have the habit of eating snacks while watching television or doing any other activity. In that case, it is advisable to put sack portions on a plate instead of eating from the package. Eating from the package will have you unconsciously overeating. Always control your snack portions.

- Whenever you are having difficulty finding healthy snacks, you should consider consulting a dietician or your health care provider for tips and ideas on how best you can make your snacks more nutritious. Implement the ideas that will work best for you and your family, and always make sure you motivate yourself to do what is right for your body.

What Constitutes a Healthy Snack?

As mentioned earlier, it may be challenging to figure out which snacks can be considered healthy. When buying your snacks, try to read the labels and find information concerning the serving size and the nutritional information. Always remember to pay particular attention to the serving size because it is usually easy to overeat and forget about portion control. Also, remember to get the appropriate serving out of the packaging and put the packet away before you start snacking so that you are not tempted to go for more. If a snack lists sugar as one of the first ingredients, avoid it.

The size of your snack should strike a balance between giving you enough calories to satisfy you and not too many calories that promote unwanted weight gain. The food that you pick should be low in added sugar and fats but high in fiber and water. That way, you stay fuller for longer yet have consumed fewer calories. The simple fact here is that an apple is definitely a healthier option than a bag of chips. Fruits, low-fat foods, and whole grains are advisable in comparison with food that is high in added sugars.

Remember that fresh fruit is a much healthier choice than a fruit-flavored drink. A snack that pairs protein and carbohydrates will keep you full for the longest time. For example, you can have vegan cheese and an apple, whole-wheat crackers with peanut butter, or simply fresh fruit and vegan plain yogurt. Fruits and vegetables are always some of the best choices you could make for snack time. They are low in calories and fat, and they are full of vitamins.

Some components that constitute a healthy snack include apples, raisins, bananas, and fruit puree without any added sugars. Carrots, nuts, whole grain dry cereal, low-fat or non-fat vegan yogurt, and pumpkin seeds are the healthiest. Always be sure to include a vegetable or fruit with each snack. You must have travel handy snack ideas for when you are on the go. Snacks that are good for the road include nuts, seeds, and fruits.

One good idea is to pack leftovers and use them as snacks. You can package leftover food into small snack-size containers that can be stored in the fridge or freezer. You must also understand the way your body reacts to your eating. You should know when you are hungry and when you are full. Understand your body's signs. Try by all means to avoid distractions when eating. Eating absent-mindedly usually results in overeating. Try as much as possible to focus on your meal or snack until you are done, ensuring that you have taken the correct portion.

The Recipes

To support what you have learned so far concerning healthy, plant-based snacks, we will outline some recipes that you can consider taking part in your recipe book. These recipes will help you add variety to your snacking time and avoid the boredom that can lead to emotional eating, binging and other forms of unhealthy eating. The nutritional variety is also enhanced. Therefore, this chapter will assist you in snacking away with some healthy dishes instead of going towards junky snacks in a bid to control your hunger.

Edamame

If one of the questions that you ask before taking a snack is, "Is it a little bit salty?" then edamame is meant for you. Edamame is a healthy salty snack whose main ingredient is soybeans. Edamame allows you to squeeze the soybeans directly from their pods into your mouth with satisfaction that nothing else can give. Edamame is super-rich in proteins.

What You Need

- Toasted sesame oil (toasted) (½ tablespoon)
- Frozen in the shell edamame pods(1 pound)
- Small garlic (1 clove)
- Kosher or fine sea salt (¾ teaspoon)
- More sea salt for the water

Instructions

1. In a large saucepan, add water and bring it to a boil. Add one teaspoon of kosher salt and the edamame to the boiling water.
2. Allow the edamame to boil for about four to five minutes until it becomes bright green and tender before draining it.
3. Place the edamame in a bowl and add the sesame oil and salt.
4. Grate the garlic clove into the bowl using a microplane.
5. Gently toss until everything is coated evenly, and break up any garlic clumps that stick together.
6. Serve the dish while it is still warm in a serving bowl and add an accompanying smaller bowl for the discarded pods.

Kale Bruschetta

This snack is perfect as an appetizer. The better part of it all is that it is a nutritious plant-based food. This recipe can make eight pieces, and it takes 25 minutes to prepare.

What You Need

- Kale (1 bunch)
- Fresh and sliced whole-grain bread (100 grams)
- Balsamic glaze
- Halved grape tomatoes (1 cup)

Instructions

1. Put water in a large pot and let it boil and medium to high heat.
2. Place the kale leaves in the water that is already boiling in the large pot.
3. Cover the pot with a lid and cook the kale leaves for about five minutes until it is tender. Drain the water.
4. Use your hands to squeeze out any extra liquid after draining so that the bread won't be soggy.
5. Prepare eight pieces of toasted bread and put them on a serving platter. Spread one tablespoon of Cannellini bean sauce on the bread.
6. Add a layer of kale on top of the Cannellini bean sauce spread. Scatter some grape tomatoes on top.
7. Generously, drizzle Balsamic glaze, and your Kale Bruschetta is ready to serve.

Hummus With Herbs

This recipe gives you a hummus that has far much lower fat content when compared to the traditional one. When humus is placed inside veggie wraps, the snack is irresistibly tasty and appetizing. You can have this dish as a topping for baked potatoes. Alternatively, you can eat it along with vegetable sticks.

What You Need

- Blanched and lightly packed, fresh basil leaves (1 cup)
- Blanched and lightly packed fresh tarragon leaves (½ cup)
- Vegetable broth (1 cup)
- Garlic (2 cloves)
- Cooked garbanzo beans (4 cups)
- Lemon juice
- Lightly packed and fresh flat-leaf parsley leaves (½ cup)
- Toasted sesame seeds (2 tablespoons)
- Chopped chives (¼ cup)

Instructions

1. Coarsely chop the basil and tarragon after patting them until they are dry
2. Put the tarragon and basil in a food processor and add the parsley, broth, beans, sesame seeds, lemon juice, and garlic.
3. Process until you achieve the desired consistency
4. Add the chives and stir well to blend them in.
5. For storage, transfer the herbed hummus into an airtight container and place it in the fridge for not more than four days.

Pea Guacamole

Pea guacamole is an excellent replacement for some dishes that require avocado. This tasty snack combines frozen green peas and add-ins such as cumin, fresh garlic, hot sauce, cilantro, and lime. Enjoy the creamy dip, an ultra-light snack that you can prepare in just 35 minutes.

What You Need

- Frozen green peas (2 cups)
- Fresh lime juice (¼ cup)
- Crushed garlic (1 teaspoon)
- Ground cumin (½ teaspoon)
- Chopped tomato (1)
- Chopped fresh cilantro (½ cup)
- Chopped green onions (4)
- Hot sauce (⅛ teaspoon)
- Sea salt

What You Need

1. Use a food processor to blend the garlic, peas, lime juice, and cumin until it is smooth.
2. Transfer the process ingredients into a bowl. Add in tomato, cilantro, green onion, and hot sauce and stir to mix. Add the salt to your preferred taste.
3. Cover the bowl and refrigerate for about 30 minutes to ensure that the flavors blend well.

Potato Pancakes

You might be familiar with potato pancakes, but you surely need to check out these ones because they are plant-based! This recipe is void of ingredients that may potentially damage your arteries by promoting the accumulation of fatty deposits. The toppings that are used in this recipe are dairy-free. You just need 50 minutes to get your plant-based potato pancakes on your table.

What You Need

- Grated russet potatoes (2)
- Large grated zucchini (1)

- Finely grated yellow onion (½)
- Oat flour (½ cup)
- Baking powder (1 teaspoon)
- Freshly ground black pepper (½ teaspoon)

Instructions

1. **Preheat your oven to 425ºF.**
2. Use parchment paper to wrap two sheet pans.
3. Spread a kitchen towel on a clean kitchen towel and spread half of the grated vegetables over the towel. Roll the kitchen towel over the vegetables and then wring it to get the extra moisture out
4. Put the wrung vegetables into a large bowl and repeat the moisture-removal process with the rest of the vegetables.
5. Add the flour, pepper, and baking powder into a small bowl and mix well. Add the mixture to the vegetables in the large mixing bowl.
6. Mix well with your hands to ensure that the flour and baking powder is evenly distributed.
7. Get about a quarter cup of the potato mixture. Use your hands to shape it into a semi-tight ball. With your palms, flatten the underside of the ball you made and place it on the prepared pan.
8. Repeat step (7) until the rest of the potato mixture is finished. Be sure to leave a distance of about to inches between the pancakes.
9. After baking for 12 minutes, flip onto the other side. Bake for 12 minutes again or until the crispiness of the pancakes becomes appealing to you.
10. Serve and use the condiments of your choice as toppings.

CONCLUSION

Weight-loss issues are gaining center stage in the lives of women, regardless of age. There are various reasons why ladies prefer to lose weight and maintain a certain number of pounds. Some do it to maintain the shape that they want, while some are pushed for health reasons. The reasons are plenty. Whatever the reasons might be, the bottom line is that women are desperate for weight-loss methods that help them lose weight and keep it off, too. Most dieting and exercising regimes that exist can appear to be working in the first few days, weeks, or months because the weight loss will be evident. Usually, the problem comes with maintaining the weight—they gain it back.

Plant-based diets have gained remarkable recognition in the health and dieting arena due to their role in sustainable weight loss. If done the right way consistently, a plant-based diet can see you losing weight for a lifetime. Many celebrities also adopted this diet for various reasons. Zac Efron, Liam Hemsworth, Venus Williams, Jay Z, and Beyonce are celebrities who now embrace plant-based diets.

Plant-based diets are defined differently, depending on personal preferences, beliefs, and reasons for undertaking the diet. Generally, four main definitions have gained popularity in the past decade. These are

- **The vegan:** In this diet, no meat or animal by-products are allowed at all. This is the type of plant-based diet that is emphasized in this book.

- **The vegetarian:** Meat is excluded, but eggs, dairy products, and seafood are allowed.

- **Whole food plant-based diet:** Processed or refined foods are prohibited in this plant-based diet.

- **Mediterranean diet:** This diet allows people to eat moderate amounts of meat and animal products.

Apart from achieving weight loss, the plant-based diet comes with many other benefits to you. Plants have essential compounds that are called phytochemicals, which exhibit various medicinal properties that are helpful to your body. One of the attributes is that some of these phytochemicals show antioxidant properties that are helpful in reducing the risks of degenerative diseases like cancers. Plant-based products are nutritionally rich. They contain macronutrients such as carbohydrates and proteins and micronutrients like calcium. Plant foods also contain large amounts of fiber.

There are health benefits that accompany consistent consumption of plant-based foods. Plant-based diets are associated with reduced instances of diabetes. The chances of being affected by conditions such as heart disease and stroke are also decreased. Scientific reports have reported the role of plant-based foods in preventing or reducing the severity of sleep apnea, constipation, cognitive decline, and some cancers such as gastrointestinal cancer.

Although foods that are originally from plants are rich in various nutrients, there are other nutrients that you cannot find in them. Examples of such nutrients are vitamin B12, creatine, carnosine, taurine, heme iron, and vitamin D3. These nutrients that are not available in plants have crucial functions in the body. For instance, carnosine is important for reducing muscle fatigue. Long-chain omega-3 polyunsaturated fatty acids are highly involved in regulating the fluidity of the cell membrane that surrounds the cells. This means that there should be other ways to get the nutrients that are unavailable in plants. Supplements are among the best possible options.

It's also important to understand how plant-based diets enhance weight loss. The fiber in plant products plays a huge role in aiding weight loss. Fiber is digested at a much slower rate in the body. This keeps the food in the digestive system for longer, thereby keeping you satiated for extended periods of time. Such a scenario reduces the temptation to overeat, and this contributes to losing weight. Plant foods also create a calorie deficit in the body.

Plants are low-calorie foods, so they do not leave the body with excess calories that can convert to fat for storage when they are digested. The energy that is stored in the form of fat contributes much to the overall weight gain of an individual. Plant-based diets also enhance insulin sensitivity. This helps to keep blood sugar levels at normal ranges. Otherwise, spikes in blood sugar levels leave the body with much more glucose to convert to fat. Scientific studies also reported that diets that are rich in plant-based foods improve the efficiency of your metabolism. The more efficient your metabolism is, the better the ability of the body to use up blood glucose and maintain it at normal levels that do not enhance weight gain.

Another important aspect is to note that losing weight through a plant-based diet is not automatic. There are things that you should take into consideration for you to lose weight successfully. For instance, if you cook your vegetables with too much cooking oil, you are more likely to gain weight due to the high-calorie content of fats. Lifestyle habits such as eating out more often can also promote weight gain, even when you are on a diet that is dominated by plant foods. Restaurants usually use high amounts of oil for cooking, and they also use methods such as deep-frying, which supports weight gain.

If you are used to an animal-based diet, switching to a plant-based diet can be challenging. To increase our chances of success, make the transition as gradual and smooth as possible. To successfully do this, follow these steps:

1. Begin by adjusting your portions so that the plant-based portions slowly take the better part of your whole meals.
2. As you increase portions of plant foods, reduce your meat consumption.
3. As time progresses, eliminate meat entirely from your diet.
4. Being able to drop meat is a great breakthrough in this transition. Now, find a substitution for animal-based products like yogurt, cheese, cream, milk, and eggs.

Once you have been able to smoothly go through the transition from an animal-based to a plant-based diet, the next thing is to sustain the diet. Avoid all processed foods, sweeteners, and animal products. Embrace variety and accommodate different types of plant-based foods in their different colors. The colors of plant-based foods are indicative of the type of nutrients that they contain. Other tips that will help include eating all meals, snacking whenever you feel hungry, eating at home more than out, as well as creating or joining support groups whose vision statements are centered on plant-based diets. Also, embrace habits that are supportive of weight loss, such as exercise and meditation.

This book ended with a variety of recipes that you can incorporate into your recipe book. All the recipes have a unique touch to your diet, taste buds, and to your ultimate aim — losing weight. It is my sincere desire that this book will help you to achieve sustainable weight loss that you can maintain in the long run without feeling bored. Go ahead and practice what you learned in this book and do away with the "try and error" methods that have clogged the internet. I wish you all the best as you lose weight the plant-based way!

Leave a 1-click Review

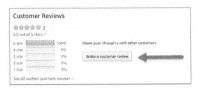

I would be incredibly <u>thankful</u> if you could take just 60 seconds to write a brief review on Amazon, even if its just a few sentences!

Just For You

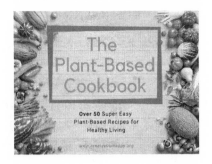

A Free Gift to My Readers
Over 50 Plant-Based Recipes. Download and Start Eating
Healthy Today!

www.createyourhappy.org/cookbook

REFERENCES

Avocado chickpea salad collard wraps. (2017, January 3). Emilie Eats. https://www.emilieeats.com/avocado-chickpea-salad-collard-wraps/

Barnard, N. D., & Leroy, F. (2020). Children and adults should avoid consuming animal products to reduce the risk for chronic disease: YES. *The American Journal of Clinical Nutrition.* https://doi.org/10.1093/ajcn/nqaa235

Beckman, J., & Design, H. (2003, December 18). *Immunity granted.* Men's Health. https://www.menshealth.com/health/a19528219/immunity-granted/

Bendich, A. (2001). Dietary reference intakes for vitamin C, vitamin E, selenium, and carotenoids institute of medicine Washington, DC: National Academy Press, 2000 ISBN: 0-309-06935-1. *Nutrition,* 17(4), 364. https://doi.org/10.1016/s0899-9007(00)00596-7

Benton, D., & Donohoe, R. (2011). The influence of creatine supplementation on the cognitive functioning of vegetarians and omnivores. *The British Journal of Nutrition, 105*(7), 1100–1105. https://doi.org/10.1017/S0007114510004733

Bravo, R. (2013, February 15). *Herbed Hummus.* Forks over Knives. https://www.forksoverknives.com/recipes/vegan-sauces-condiments/herbed-hummus/

Chiu, T. H. T., Pan, W.-H., Lin, M.-N., & Lin, C.-L. (2018). Vegetarian diet, change in dietary patterns, and diabetes risk: a prospective study. *Nutrition & Diabetes, 8*(1). https://doi.org/10.1038/s41387-018-0022-4

Coyle, D. (2018, October 3). *Starchy vs. Non-Starchy Vegetables: Food lists and nutrition facts.* Healthline; Healthline Media. https://www.healthline.com/nutrition/starchy-vs-non-starchy-vegetables

Davidson, K. (2021, May 10). *20 Tasty fruits with health benefits.* Healthline. https://www.healthline.com/nutrition/healthy-fruit

Donahue, A. (2019). *3 reasons you're not losing weight on a plant-based diet.* MamaSezz. https://www.mamasezz.com/blogs/news/3-reasons-youre-not-losing-weight-on-a-plant-based-diet

Esselstyn, A., & Esselstyn, J. (2015, June 28). *Kale bruschetta recipe.* Forks over Knives. https://www.forksoverknives.com/recipes/vegan-snacks-appetizers/kale-bruschetta/

Exploring Opinions on plant-based eating. (n.d.). Sous Vide Guy. https://sousvideguy.com/exploring-opinions-plant-based-eating/

Forer, B. (2011, April 15). *Weight loss improves memory, research reveals.* ABC News. https://abcnews.go.com/Health/weight-loss-improves-memory-research-reveals/story?id=13383600

Fox, H. (2020, July 31). *Vegan chickpea curry recipe – Ready in just 25 minutes!* https://hurrythefoodup.com/vegan-chickpea-curry-ready/

Gilmour, L. (2018, May 31). *Ariana Grande on being neighbors with Miley and loving all things British.* Mirror. https://www.mirror.co.uk/3am/celebrity-news/ariana-grande-i-love-animals-4754625

Gröber, U., Kisters, K., & Schmidt, J. (2013). Neuroenhancement with vitamin b12—underestimated neurological significance. *Nutrients, 5*(12), 5031–5045. https://doi.org/10.3390/nu5125031

Gunnars, K. (2018, July 24). *Mediterranean diet 101: A meal plan and beginner's guide.* Healthline. https://www.healthline.com/nutrition/mediterranean-diet-meal-plan

Hall, K. D., Guo, J., Courville, A. B., Boring, J., Brychta, R., Chen, K. Y., Darcey, V., Forde, C. G., Gharib, A. M., Gallagher, I., Howard, R., Joseph, P. V., Milley, L., Ouwerkerk, R., Raisinger, K., Rozga, I., Schick, A., Stagliano, M., Torres, S., & Walter, M. (2021a). Effect of a plant-based, low-fat diet versus an animal-based, ketogenic diet on ad libitum energy intake. *Nature Medicine.* https://doi.org/10.1038/s41591-020-01209-1

Hall, K. D., Guo, J., Courville, A. B., Boring, J., Brychta, R., Chen, K. Y., Darcey, V., Forde, C. G., Gharib, A. M., Gallagher, I., Howard, R., Joseph, P. V., Milley, L., Ouwerkerk, R., Raisinger, K., Rozga, I., Schick, A., Stagliano, M., Torres, S., & Walter, M. (2021b). Effect of a plant-based, low-fat diet versus an animal-based, ketogenic diet on ad libitum energy intake. *Nature Medicine, 27*, 344–353. https://doi.org/10.1038/s41591-020-01209-1

Harvard School of Public Health. (2018, August 20). *Vegetables and fruits.* The Nutrition Source. https://www.hsph.harvard.edu/nutritionsource/what-should-you-eat/vegetables-and-fruits/

Heger, E. (2020, October 28). *10 benefits of losing weight: How shedding just 5% of your body weight may improve your blood sugar, self-esteem, and sex drive.* Insider. https://www.insider.com/benefits-of-losing-weight

Holick, M. F., Binkley, N. C., Bischoff-Ferrari, H. A., Gordon, C. M., Hanley, D. A., Heaney, R. P., Murad, M. H., Weaver, C. M., & Endocrine Society. (2011). Evaluation, treatment, and prevention of vitamin D deficiency: an Endocrine Society clinical practice guideline. *The Journal of Clinical Endocrinology and Metabolism*, 96(7), 1911–1930. https://doi.org/10.1210/jc.2011-0385

House, B. T., Cook, L. T., Gyllenhammer, L. E., Schraw, J. M., Goran, M. I., Spruijt-Metz, D., Weigensberg, M. J., & Davis, J. N. (2013). Meal skipping is linked to increased visceral adipose tissue and triglycerides in overweight minority youth. *Obesity*, 22(5), E77–E84. https://doi.org/10.1002/oby.20487

independent.co.uk. (2017, August 10). *Why you should stop eating meat immediately.* The Independent. https://www.independent.co.uk/life-style/food-and-drink/why-british-people-eat-less-meat-reasons-health-weight-environment-ethics-vegan-vegetarian-a7886076.html

Jiang, X., Huang, J., Song, D., Deng, R., Wei, J., & Zhang, Z. (2017). Increased consumption of fruit and vegetables is related to a reduced risk of cognitive impairment and dementia: Meta-analysis. *Frontiers in Aging Neuroscience*, 9. https://doi.org/10.3389/fnagi.2017.00018

Kahleova, H., Petersen, K. F., Shulman, G. I., Alwarith, J., Rembert, E., Tura, A., Hill, M., Holubkov, R., & Barnard, N. D. (2020). Effect of a low-fat vegan diet on body weight, insulin sensitivity, postprandial metabolism, and intramyocellular and hepatocellular lipid levels in overweight adults. *JAMA Network*

Open, 3(11), e2025454. https://doi.org/10.1001/jamanetworkopen.2020.25454

Kaitlin. (2016, November 16). *Lentil vegetable soup*. The Garden Grazer. https://www.thegardengrazer.com/lentil-vegetable-soup/

Kannan, D. (2020, December 14). *Find the right balance: Here's why a good dinner is important for health and wellbeing*. https://yourstory.com/weekender/dinner-health-diet-vegetables-spices-balance/amp

Kate. (2018, March 26). *Green pea quinoa (vegan, gluten-free)*. The Green Loot. https://thegreenloot.com/green-pea-quinoa-vegan/

Kate. (2020, July 14). *Vegan Mediterranean quinoa salad with chickpeas*. The Green Loot. https://thegreenloot.com/vegan-mediterranean-quinoa-salad/

Kay, S. (2018, August 9). *Why you should avoid artificial sweeteners*. Stephanie Kay | Nutritionist & Speaker. https://kaynutrition.com/avoid-artificial-sweeteners/

Kern, B. D., & Robinson, T. L. (2011). Effects of β-alanine supplementation on performance and body composition in collegiate wrestlers and football players. *Journal of Strength and Conditioning Research*, 25(7), 1804–1815. https://doi.org/10.1519/JSC.0b013e3181e741cf

Khorsandi, H., Nikpayam, O., Yousefi, R., Parandoosh, M., Hosseinzadeh, N., Saidpour, A., & Ghorbani, A. (2019). Zinc supplementation improves body weight management, inflammatory biomarkers and insulin resistance in individuals with obesity: a randomized, placebo-controlled, double-blind trial. *Diabetology & Metabolic Syndrome*, 11(1). https://doi.org/10.1186/s13098-019-0497-8

Krans, B. (2020). *Almond Milk versus Cow's Milk versus Soy Milk versus Rice Milk.* Healthline. https://www.healthline.com/health/milk-almond-cow-soy-rice

Lawler, M. (2019, October 7). *Beginner's guide to a plant-based diet: Food list, meal plan, benefits, and more.* everydayhealth.com. https://www.everydayhealth.com/diet-nutrition/plant-based-diet-food-list-meal-plan-benefits-more/

Leafyplace.com. (2019a, June 6). *27 types of berries: List of berries with their picture and name.* Leafy Place. https://leafyplace.com/types-of-berries/

lettucevegout.com. (n.d.). *Herbs and spices for a balanced vegan diet: How to eat more as a vegan.* Lettuce Veg Out. https://lettucevegout.com/vegan-food-groups/herbs-spices/

lettucevegout.com. (2019, March 21). *Why it's important to eat leafy green vegetables, especially for vegans.* lettuce Veg Out. https://lettucevegout.com/nutrition/leafy-green-vegetables-vegans/

loveandlemons.com. (2017, March 28). *Best Buddha bowl.* Love and Lemons. https://www.loveandlemons.com/buddha-bowl-recipe/

loveandlemons.com. (2016, July 13). *Stuffed poblano peppers.* Love and Lemons. https://www.loveandlemons.com/stuffed-poblano-peppers/

loveandlemons.com. (2017, November 1). *Vegan broccoli soup.* Love and Lemons. https://www.loveandlemons.com/vegan-broccoli-soup/

loveandlemons.com. (2018, January 15). *Adzuki bean bowls.* Love and Lemons. https://www.loveandlemons.com/adzuki-beans-recipe/

loveandlemons.com. (2019a, May 13). *Sesame soba noodles.* Love and Lemons. https://www.loveandlemons.com/sesame-soba-noodles/

loveandlemons.com. (2019b, October 10). *Easy vegetarian chili recipe.* Love and Lemons. https://www.loveandlemons.com/vegetarian-chili-recipe/

loveandlemons.com. (2020, June 7). *Radish salad.* Love and Lemons. https://www.loveandlemons.com/radish-salad/

Lukaszuk, J. M., Robertson, R. J., Arch, J. E., Moore, G. E., Yaw, K. M., Kelley, D. E., Rubin, J. T., & Moyna, N. M. (2002). Effect of creatine supplementation and a lacto-ovo-vegetarian diet on muscle creatine concentration. *International Journal of Sports Nutrition and Exercise Metabolism, 12*(3), 336–348. https://doi.org/10.1123/ijsnem.12.3.336

MacKeen, D. (2021, May 18). *Why the plant milk in your coffee may not be as healthy as you think.* The Irish Times. https://www.irishtimes.com/life-and-style/food-and-drink/why-the-plant-milk-in-your-coffee-may-not-be-as-healthy-as-you-think-1.4564362

Mae, K. (2014, December 11). *Healthy potato pancakes recipe.* Forks over Knives. https://www.forksoverknives.com/recipes/vegan-breakfast/potato-pancakes/

Malar, D., & Devi, K. (2014). Dietary polyphenols for treatment of Alzheimer's disease– future research and development. *Current Pharmaceutical Biotechnology, 15*(4), 330–342. https://doi.org/10.2174/1389201015666140813122703

Mayo Clinic Staff. (2017). *The whole truth about whole grains.* Mayo Clinic. https://www.mayoclinic.org/healthy-lifestyle/nutrition-and-healthy-eating/in-depth/whole-grains/art-20047826

Mayo Clinic Staff. (2019, June 21). *Mediterranean diet: A heart-healthy eating plan*. Mayo Clinic. https://www.mayoclinic.org/healthy-lifestyle/nutrition-and-healthy-eating/in-depth/mediterranean-diet/art-20047801

mayo clinic health system. (2017, January 3). *Processed foods that you should know*. www.mayoclinichealthsystem.org. https://www.mayoclinichealthsystem.org/hometown-health/speaking-of-health/processed-foods-what-you-should-know

McDermott, A. (2018, December 3). *Everything you need to know about stevia*. Healthline; Healthline Media. https://www.healthline.com/health/food-nutrition/stevia-side-effects

McDougall, M. (2015, April 1). *Green pea guacamole recipe*. Forks over Knives. https://www.forksoverknives.com/recipes/vegan-snacks-appetizers/pea-guacamole/

McMacken, M., & Shah, S. (2017). A plant-based diet for the prevention and treatment of type 2 diabetes. *Journal of Geriatric Cardiology: JGC, 14*(5), 342–354. https://doi.org/10.11909/j.issn.1671-5411.2017.05.009

Momen, M. A. (n.d.). *Importance of dinner for a healthy life*. https://theworldbook.org/importance-of-dinner/

Nast, C. (2018, March 19). *Zac Efron's newest friend is a tiger shark*. Teen Vogue. https://www.teenvogue.com/story/zac-efron-shares-his-grooming-routine-and-life-advice

National Institutes of Health. (2018, July 9). *Intensive weight loss helps knee arthritis*. National Institutes of Health (NIH). https://www.nih.gov/news-events/nih-research-matters/intensive-weight-loss-helps-knee-arthritis

Nemours Kidshealth. (n.d.). *Vegetarian diets (for parents)*. Kidshealth.org. https://kidshealth.org/en/parents/vegetarianism.html%20/t%20_blank

NHS Choices. (2018, August 2). *Eat well*. NHS. https://www.nhs.uk/live-well/eat-well/the-vegan-diet/

NHS Choices. (2019). *Eat well*. NHS. https://www.nhs.uk/live-well/eat-well/what-are-processed-foods/

Overhisa, S. (2020, February 25). *Easy edamame*. A Couple Cooks. https://www.acouplecooks.com/easy-edamame/

peta.org. (2010, July 7). *Don't we need to eat meat and dairy products to be healthy?* PETA. https://www.peta.org/about-peta/faq/dont-we-need-to-eat-meat-and-dairy-products-to-be-healthy/

Physicians Committee for Responsible Medicine. (2019). *Weight loss*. Physicians Committee for Responsible Medicine. https://www.pcrm.org/health-topics/weight-loss

Piatt, J. (2017). *This cheese is nuts! : Delicious vegan cheese at home*. Avery, An Imprint Of Penguin Random House.

Pike, A. (2019, February 7). *The Basics of a vegan diet*. IFIC Foundation. https://foodinsight.org/basics-of-vegan-diet/

Poore, J., & Nemecek, T. (2018). Reducing food's environmental impacts through producers and consumers. *Science, 360*(6392), 987–992. https://doi.org/10.1126/science.aaq0216

provitamil.com. (2010). *The Importance of Eating Lunch: Great tasting, non-dairy alternatives to milk & soya*. Provitamil.com. https://www.provitamil.com/healthier-lifestyle/the-importance-of-eating-lunch.htm

Rae, C., Digney, A. L., McEwan, S. R., & Bates, T. C. (2003). Oral creatine monohydrate supplementation improves brain performance: a double-blind, placebo-controlled, cross–over trial. *Proceedings of the Royal Society of London. Series B: Biological Sciences, 270*(1529), 2147–2150. https://doi.org/10.1098/rspb.2003.2492

Richards, L. (2021, August 24). *Is plant-based meat healthy? Pros and cons.* www.medicalnewstoday.com. https://www.medical-newstoday.com/articles/is-plant-based-meat-healthy#is-it-healthy

Rush, J. (2020, September 17). *Vegan-loaded sweet potatoes.* Rescue Dog Kitchen. https://www.rescuedogkitchen.com/vegan-loaded-sweet-potatoes/

Schlesinger, S., Ballon, A., & Neuenschwander, M. (2018). Skipping breakfast and risk of type 2 diabetes: A systematic review and meta-analysis of prospective studies. *Revue d'Épidémiologie et de Santé Publique, 66,* S352. https://doi.org/10.1016/j.respe.2018.05.314

Scott-Thomas, C. (2015, March 16). *Health or ethics? Reason for a vegan diet may affect health outcomes.* Foodnavigator.com. https://www.foodnavigator.com/Article/2015/03/16/Health-or-ethics-Reason-for-vegan-diet-may-affect-health-outcomes

Shivaraj, M. C., Marcy, G., Low, G., Ryu, J. R., Zhao, X., Rosales, F. J., & Goh, E. L. K. (2012). Taurine induces proliferation of neural stem cells and synapse development in the developing mouse brain. *PLoS ONE, 7*(8), e42935. https://doi.org/10.1371/journal.pone.0042935

Smith, A. (2020, April 27). *Vegan diet: Health benefits, risks, and meal tips.* www.medicalnewstoday.com. https://www.medicalnewstoday.com/articles/149636

Spritzler, F. (2016). *11 reasons why berries are among the healthiest foods on earth.* Healthline. https://www.healthline.com/nutrition/11-reasons-to-eat-berries

Streit, L. (2019, September 10). *Vegetarian diet for weight loss: Food list and meal plan.* Healthline. https://www.healthline.com/nutrition/vegetarian-weight-loss

Tantamango-Bartley, Y., Jaceldo-Siegl, K., Fan, J., & Fraser, G. (2012). Vegetarian diets and the incidence of cancer in a low-risk population. *Cancer Epidemiology Biomarkers & Prevention*, 22(2), 286–294. https://doi.org/10.1158/1055-9965.epi-12-1060

Tran, E., Dale, H. F., Jensen, C., & Lied, G. A. (2020). Effects of plant-based diets on weight status: A systematic review. *Diabetes, Metabolic Syndrome and Obesity: Targets and Therapy*, Volume 13, 3433–3448. https://doi.org/10.2147/dmso.s272802

Vegan Health & Evidence-Based Nutrient Recommendations. (n.d.). *Omega-3s*. VeganHealth.org. https://veganhealth.org/omega-3s/

Vincent, H. K., Bourguignon, C. M., & Taylor, A. G. (2010). Relationship of the dietary phytochemical index to weight gain, oxidative stress, and inflammation in overweight young adults. *Journal of Human Nutrition and Dietetics*, 23(1), 20–29. https://doi.org/10.1111/j.1365-277x.2009.00987.x

Virtues, V. (2016, April 26). *6 qualities of people who never quit*. Addicted 2 Success. https://addicted2success.com/success-advice/6-qualities-of-people-who-never-quit/

Vitoria Miñana, I. (2017). The nutritional limitations of plant-based beverages in infancy and childhood. *Nutrición Hospitalaria*. https://doi.org/10.20960/nh.931

Vogel, K. (2021, April 28). *Plant-based and loving it! Here are 50 celebrities who went vegan (and might inspire you to do the same)*. Parade: Entertainment, Recipes, Health, Life, Holidays. https://parade.com/1198380/kaitlin-vogel/vegan-celebrities/

Wang, H.-X. . (2002). Vitamin B12, folate, and Alzheimer's disease. *Drug Development Research*, 56(2), 111–122. https://doi.org/10.1002/ddr.10066

webmd.com. (2019). *Macular degeneration*. WebMD. https://www.webmd.com/eye-health/macular-degeneration/default.htm

webmd.com. (2020). *Difference between starchy and non-starchy vegetables*. WebMD. https://www.webmd.com/diet/difference-between-starchy-non-starchy-vegetables

Weil, A. (2011). *How much vitamin k for strong bones?*. DrWeil.com. https://www.drweil.com/vitamins-supplements-herbs/vitamins/how-much-vitamin-k-for-strong-bones/